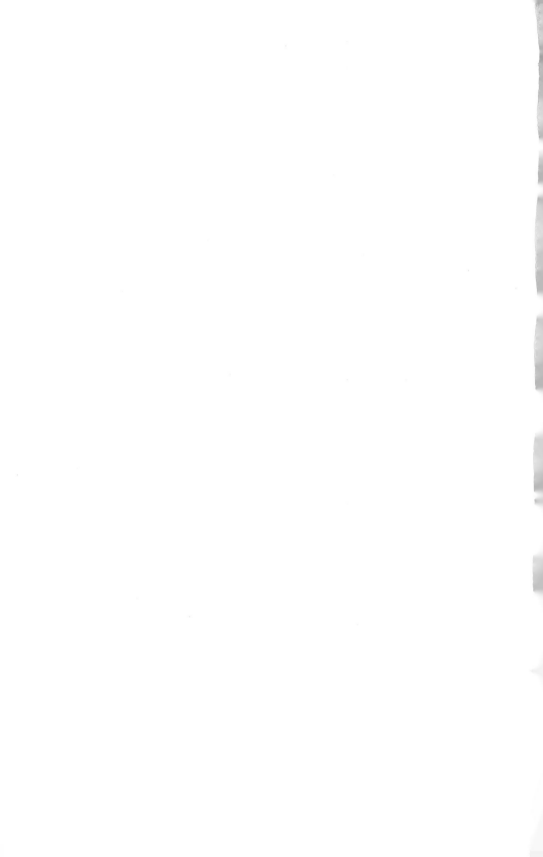

PSYCHODYNAMIC PRACTICE
IN A MANAGED CARE ENVIRONMENT

PSYCHODYNAMIC PRACTICE IN A MANAGED CARE ENVIRONMENT

A Strategic Guide for Clinicians

Michael B. Sperling
Amy Sack
Charles L. Field

THE GUILFORD PRESS
New York   London

©2000 The Guilford Press
A Division of Guilford Publications, Inc.
72 Spring Street, New York, NY 10012
www.guilford.com

Printed in the United States of America

This book is printed on acid-free paper.

Last digit is print number: 9 8 7 6 5 4 3 2 1

Library of Congress Cataloging-in-Publication Data

Sperling, Michael B.
  Psychodynamic practice in a managed care environment :
a strategic guide for clinicians / Michael B. Sperling, Amy
Sack, Charles L. Field.
     p. cm.
  Includes bibliographical references and index.
  ISBN 1-57230-133-3
  1. Psychodynamic psychotherapy—Effect of managed care
on. I. Sack, Amy. II. Field, Charles Lawrence, 1957–
III. Title.
  [DNLM: 1. Psychoanalytic Therapy. 2. Documentation—
methods. 3. Managed Care Programs. 4. Psychotherapy,
Brief—methods. WM 460.6 S749p 1999]
  RC489.P72 S66   1999
  616.89′14—dc21   99-048197
                                                              CIP

About the Authors

Michael B. Sperling, PhD, is Acting Dean of University College, as well as Professor of Psychology at Fairleigh Dickinson University in Teaneck, New Jersey. His research and clinical interests include adult attachment and love relations, character pathology, psychodynamic psychotherapy, and family therapy. He has published numerous scholarly journal articles, and edited *Attachment in Adults: Clinical and Developmental Perspectives,* with William H. Berman (Guilford Press, 1994). Dr. Sperling serves as a board member for the Psychoanalytic Research Society of the Division of Psychoanalysis of the American Psychological Association, and is a Council of Fellows Executive Committee member of the American Council on Education.

Dr. Sperling completed a postdoctoral psychology fellowship at the New York Hospital–Cornell Medical Center in White Plains, New York, and an American Council on Education Fellowship in academic administration at Baruch College of the City University of New York.

Amy Sack, PhD, is a clinical psychologist and currently an MBA candidate at the Yale University School of Management. Most recently, she served as an associate in the Computer Science Corporation's Health Care Group. She formerly worked as a psychologist in the Women's Trauma Program of Elmcrest Hospital in Portland, Connecticut, and she has published journal articles on the subject of borderline psychopathology and attachment theory.

Charles L. Field, PhD, is a clinical psychologist in private practice in South Windsor, Connecticut. Dr. Field works with children, adolescents, adults, couples, and families. He is dedicated to helping people create and discover meaning in their lives. He is especially interested in identifying and overcoming the obstacles that hinder people from experiencing hope, responsibility toward self and others, and personal freedom.

Acknowledgments

This book, like most, was conceived and written in a rather circuitous creative process. That psychodynamic therapy and managed care are difficult to integrate under the best of circumstances has made the project even more labyrinthine. We ventured into some unproductive and discouraging areas, but having done so we also enriched our knowledge immeasurably. We have learned from and with each other, and hope that readers will also learn from and with our material.

At the start, we want to acknowledge the insightfulness, honesty, patience, and good humor we have experienced with each other. Working through this material together has not been an easy process, yet ultimately it has been a very rewarding one. We also want to thank Kitty Moore, our editor at The Guilford Press, who has herself demonstrated abundant patience with and commitment to this project.

We each give our individual acknowledgments in the following three paragraphs:

For M. B. S., family and close friends are the foundation that enables creative work to take place. My wife, Priscilla, and my daughters, Katie and Charlotte, mean everything to me.

For A. S., the following friends and family have provided the support and patience that were essential to me in the writing of this book. I would first like to acknowledge my father, Joshua Sack, MD, for his steadfast support and encouragement. I would like to express my heartfelt appreciation to Meredith Gould, PhD, for providing me with a secure base and giving me the courage to grow. I am indebted to Nancy Krim, MA, MFA, for teaching me to write and sharing her world. Special thanks to Cheryl Strauss and Elanna Pollack for their friendship and to Dustin Gordon, PhD, who made graduate school bearable. I owe a debt of gratitude to my educators, Judith Kaufman, PhD, and M. Elizabeth Langell, PhD, for facilitating my professional growth. Finally I would like to thank Thelma Jones, MD, for making the effort and Michelle Sack for being my sister.

For C. L. F., thank you, Isaac, for your love and support, and to all my patients, thank you for your collaboration.

Contents

INTRODUCTION

The Dilemmas
of Managed Care

In a relatively short period of time, managed care has become an amazingly potent entity in American health care, with approximately three-quarters market penetration. Although we cannot predict its longevity, all signs indicate that it will institutionalize even further as an inevitable way of doing business. That this situation presents both patients and clinicians with dilemmas is, by now, old news. What isn't old news is the need to pay serious attention to the conceptual and practical ways in which managed care becomes uniquely challenging for psychodynamic clinicians. That many view managed care and psychodynamic technique as incompatible represents a prevailing sensibility that has led to the paucity of serious attention. Yet, in contrast to this is the reality that many psychodynamic clinicians nonetheless do currently work with managed care and many others are interested in learning more about it.

Managed care is an inflammatory phrase. It evokes fears and experiences of dishonest and unethical treatment, breaches of confidentiality, and the destruction of the transferential foundation of many psychodynamic therapies. In addition, it elicits images of practices folding and referrals drying

1

up. Some even suggest that it's heretical to do business with the "evils" of managed care. This attitude is well founded. After all, instances of poor judgment and harmful utilization review decisions are rampant (Miller, 1996), and quality of care can be compromised (Dana, Conner, & Allen, 1996; Seligman & Levant, 1998). Additionally, the erosion of confidentiality and privacy alone can prompt a decision not to serve on any panels where patient information will be shared with a third party—and such a situation is virtually omnipresent in the managed care world (Bollas & Sundelson, 1996).

Our stance is that psychodynamics and managed care can be effectively integrated with certain patients and under certain conditions. Further, managed care is a current reality in health care which, although manifesting with many negative consequences, is at root a financially driven management technique that needs to be negotiated with on an individual level while it is responded to and challenged on legislative and regulatory levels. We have much sympathy for the powerful and justified distrust that exists toward managed care, as we see far too many ethical and clinical problems to support managed care as it exists today. These unethical and clinical challenges leave the practicing psychodynamic psychotherapist in a predicament, because the therapist who decides to have nothing to do with managed care is the same therapist who is then unavailable to work with untold numbers of potential patients. Thus it is the patient, that is, the consumer, who loses out when psychodynamic clinicians are minimally available to him/her. For this reason we think it is important to examine how we can best operate within the managed care environment as we simultaneously work to reduce its destructive impact.

As psychodynamic clinicians we have numerous tensions with which we must contend (e.g., managed care's focus on symptom reduction rather than character change), so as to provide "good enough" service to our managed care patients. We operate by the principle that we must do our best in less than ideal conditions to continue to help those who can benefit from our services. Thus, we will inevitably face dilemmas that force us to choose between the lesser among potentially harmful situations. A brief example illustrates this point:

A woman calls a therapist. She reminds the therapist that she had been a patient of his 5 years ago and also tells him that despite the advances she made in her therapy, a very upsetting event has now transpired. The woman then says that she is divorced and can no longer afford the private indemnity insurance she had previously. She tells him that she has group insurance as a state employee. She asks the therapist if he takes X (e.g., Blue Cross Blue Shield), an insurance that is case managed. She explains that all state plans are now in the hands of managed care, a change forced on all employees in the past year (a situation which has occurred in many states). She then says that she knows that X does not reimburse much but would really appreciate his time since he is one of the few people whom she trusts. The therapist listens and remembers the woman, her history of abuse, her tenacity, and her cautiousness. The therapist then considers his options and hers.

Though the above scenario is less extreme than many, it reflects both the commitment we have toward patients who return for additional treatment following termination, as well as the dilemma of considering treatment provision under less than optimal financial and, by extension, ethical circumstances. As practitioners, we have a duty not to abandon our patients. Further, no matter what our economic or philosophical position, it is clear that the party who has the most to lose and who will most suffer by the policies of managed care is the actual or potential patient. What seems clear is that in the absence of other intervening factors, this woman would be best served by her previous therapist, even if just for an extended consultation.

PSYCHODYNAMIC CONCEPTUAL FOUNDATION UNDER MANAGED CARE

We write this book from a foundation of our abiding respect for psychodynamic theory and technique, and our wish that those who share our devotion to this way of understanding and helping people will continue to meet the managed care challenge head on. When Sigmund Freud, in the face of criticisms, took psychoanalysis out of the university setting and established freestanding institutes, it was a questionable move. Many have argued that the isolationism this caused has been unfortunate, and that it has enhanced the intellectual rifts and distrusts between psychodynamics and other forms of psychotherapeutic practice. We see a similar dilemma, in the economic realm, facing psychoanalysis today, as reflected in the fact that some clinicians advocate for the complete abandonment of any claim to third-party reimbursement or negotiation with managed care. This might result in a marginalization of psychodynamics from the rest of the mental health field, exacerbating the fragility of those bridges that do already exist. We think such an approach would ultimately be hurtful. And there may even be more leverage today to advocate for psychodynamic psychotherapy's inclusion in managed care than there was a decade ago.

It seems that managed care is now in a transition from the days of "revolutionary" cost savings and seemingly unlimited growth. Managed care's growth has finally decelerated, albeit with enormous existing penetration, and many organizations are coming under critical financial and legislative scrutiny. Patients' bills of rights are being considered in several states, and national regulatory legislation is a hot-button political issue. The prohibitions on patients' malpractice suits toward HMO's are under attack, and there is the sense that managed care must police itself better or politicians and the courts will do it for them. All of this activity means that managed care is likely to be (relatively) more responsive to efforts to work collaboratively, as well as less effective in fighting challenges and stonewalling opponents. Managed care and psychodynamics appear to be less incompatible at present than at any time in the past 10 years.

Contrary to a belief held by many, the same psychodynamic conceptual foundation within which a clinician already operates can be used with many managed care patients. (We address the critical issue of what patients this applies to in Chapter Three.) While there is no need to abandon psychodynamics, we see eight fundamental differences between doing psychodynamic treatment within a managed care environment, on the one hand, and conducting a traditional (and more desirable) independent psychodynamic psychotherapy, on the other:

1. In a managed care psychodynamic approach there is typically little opportunity for a transference analysis paradigm to contextualize the work, given the time and goal constraints. Extratherapeutic transferences, however, can be used as a focus of the treatment process, and analysis of therapist–patient transference enactments can be used in an occasional, circumscribed way. This places the work more within a psychodynamic supportive framework than a psychoanalytic insight-oriented orientation.

2. Rather than addressing many aspects of character and adaptive functioning simultaneously, the choice is made to work with only one or two in any given course of therapy. In this sense the goals of supportive psychodynamic psychotherapy within managed care parallel the scope and specificity of goals that one might generate in a brief dynamic therapy, leaving out ego-confrontational techniques used in many brief therapies. In a managed care approach, patients may return to you for follow-up treatment at various times to address a current area of conflict.

3. Even while still adhering to a psychodynamic conceptual framework, communication regarding the treatment to a managed care organization is formulated mainly in an alternative functional language, with roots in behavioral and cognitive theory, that can be more readily understood by those not trained in psychodynamics.

4. Given the need for active communication with managed care organizations, the practice of privileged communication between patient and therapist is altered. There is the explicit understanding from the beginning of therapy that the patient will be periodically engaged in a treatment review and planning process, and that material for authorization will be presented to the managed care treatment reviewers.

5. The need for documentation of therapeutic work to gain authorization for further treatment requires a significant (nonreimbursed) time commitment, which is different from the traditional (and increasingly uncommon) system of submitting only a letterhead bill for reimbursement without prior authorization.

6. As with most short-term dynamic psychotherapy models, resistance needs to be worked with quickly and intensively if it is clinically indicated as a treatment focus. This is unlike tradi-

tional dynamic psychotherapy, where resistance can emerge over time and be confronted on a more selective basis.

7. Given the reality of ongoing treatment review, terminations may need to be conducted on relatively short notice when authorization is not renewed. Even if the treatment is authorized for a relatively long period, patient awareness of eventual termination remains especially present from the beginning of therapy, as it represents *the* working construct communicated by the managed care organization.

8. The focus of many treatments will be dynamically educative rather than curative. For patients who present with long-standing and/or characterological conflict areas, and who have had little prior treatment, the therapy will give them a brief experience of a depth approach. The desirable outcome is that they hold onto this and continue exploration, on their own, and in future therapies.

These differences are considerable and require much forethought in order to negotiate them effectively. Currently, the overwhelming majority of managed care systems do not recognize psychoanalysis proper and provide virtually no backing for intensive insight-oriented (transference-based) psychoanalytic psychotherapy (Pollack, 1996). And while there may be reimbursement for supportive psychodynamic psychotherapy, many patients will still not be authorized for the type of treatment that would prove most beneficial (Dana et al., 1996).

OUTLINE OF THIS BOOK

This book is written so that it can be useful either in its entirety or in parts. For psychodynamic clinicians largely unfamiliar with managed care, reading the whole book will provide the basic information for operating in a managed care environment. For those already knowledgeable about managed care, reading selected chapters may be sufficient. In any case, we have tried to make the material strategic, informative, easily readable, based on sound psychodynamic theory and research, and supportive of the field of psychodynamics.

Working within managed care adds a new and unusual element to psychodynamic treatment that makes it essentially a working triad rather than a dyad. Chapter One addresses the clinical implications of this new triadic relationship. To be able to "manage" managed care, familiarity with its motivation, politics, and structure is essential. Chapter Two presents such issues as the ways in which psychodynamic clinicians can work with managed care organizations, and the potential intellectual, financial, and ethical implications of gaining access to managed care provider networks. Chapter Three continues this discussion by focusing on the pervasive notion of medical necessity in managed care and how psychodynamic clinicians can present cases for authorization given varying combinations of functional and intrapsychic disturbance.

If you decide to have some interaction with managed care organizations, familiarity with the means to document and support your psychodynamic work is essential. The next two chapters offer clinicians some guiding principles for facilitating communication with managed care companies. Chapter Four addresses the areas of commonality between the "language" of psychodynamics and that of a functional approach. There are many areas of conceptual and linguistic overlap between "functional adaptation," its behavioral and cognitive corollaries, and psychoanalysis that are essential to be aware of in effectively communicating about one's psychodynamic work. Chapter Five applies these conceptual and linguistic understandings to the process of documenting psychodynamic work in treatment reports to managed care organizations. We present examples of write-ups that are both consistent with psychodynamic technique and readily understandable to a managed care organization.

When working with managed care, most treatments are necessarily short term, yet not all short-term psychodynamic treatments are equivalent. There are many variations in terms of time frame, elements of confrontation, and attention to transference dynamics, to name a few. Chapter Six briefly attends to these variations and their implications for psychodynamic work under managed care. Chapter Seven turns attention toward a selective annotated sampling of assessment measures, particularly those that have impact on the practice of psychodynamic treatment in a managed care environment. Those measures reviewed can be easily integrated into a clinician's office practice and, when used systematically, can serve both as a clinical tool and as a substantive means to support the efficacy of one's clinical work.

Finally, the managed care environment in mental health is a changing domain. Clinicians need to be looking ahead, not just maintaining a current position, in order to prosper financially and intellectually. Chapter Eight addresses several frequently asked questions as well as trends in managed care, offering informed speculations regarding which of these trends are likely to emerge in the coming years. Additionally, three appendices cover topics of relevance: an annotated bibliography that samples many current and useful writings on managed care that clinicians may want to read for further information; a listing of commercial test, supply, and software publishers cited in this book; and a glossary of health care and health insurance terms.

By design, this is a rather brief book. We operate from the sensibility that while psychoanalysis is an enormously intricate theory, its application in specific areas of psychodynamic technique can be relatively simple. The current mental health care environment demands flexibility and critical decision making in its application. We hope that you will find this book to be easily and quickly accessible: "brief" and "expedient" are not bad things when applied appropriately and judiciously, and are among several available choices.

After reading this book, you should be better able to:

• Navigate within managed care organizations. The goals of health care providers and insurance companies can be complementary, not necessarily antithetical. The material in this book will familiarize you with managed care provider structures and demonstrate how psychodynamic clinicians can increase their likelihood of securing treatment authorization.

• Communicate effectively with managed care organizations. Communication barriers are a large part of the problem between psychodynamic clinicians and managed care entities. This book will help you to bridge this gap and more effectively communicate and document your work in a language that is accessible to managed care and remains consistent with psychodynamic principles.

• Identify useful treatment outcome measures for your own practice. Integration of outcome measures in psychodynamic practice can be of much clinical and marketing utility. This book will present several questionnaire measures uniquely helpful to psychodynamic clinicians in their private practices.

• Respond to managed care neither out of naive fear nor with contempt, but from an informed stance, whether positive or negative. Most psychodynamic clinicians are either afraid of or hostile toward managed care. Both of these attitudes poorly position you to work in a mental health environment increasingly dominated by managed care. In order to work within and, when appropriate, advocate against managed care entities, psychodynamic clinicians must, to loosely paraphrase the first flexible treatment provider in our field (i.e., Freud), bring [managed care] insight into consciousness from the unconscious.

1

Clinical Implications
of the New Treatment Triad

Considering how to work psychodynamically with managed care
first and foremost necessitates examining how managed care is
experienced by both patient and therapist. In examining this
clinical impact, we must first consider the implications of the
new treatment situation, which is no longer a dyadic system.
(Nor is it with any third-party reimbursement system, though traditional indemnity plans certainly do not interfere with or intervene in the treatment process nearly as much.) As such, *the treatment between the therapeutic dyad now occurs in a context of two other
dyads (patient–managed care and therapist–managed care) and a triad
(patient–therapist–managed care). Psychodynamically, this means that
all those issues of dependency, authority, privacy, and the like will now
need to be understood in these other three contexts in order to potentiate
the treatment of the patient.* Thus, it is not only, for example, the
patient's pre-Oedipal and Oedipal scenarios the therapist must
consider in relation to him/herself, but also in relation to how
the managed care entity is experienced by the patient. Similarly,
the therapist must not only consider his/her countertransference experience in relation to the patient but also in relation to
the managed care reviewer. Indeed, *the therapist's responses and re-*

11

actions to managed care often are more intense (and therefore may affect the therapeutic work more) than the patient's. And both therapist and patient must consider managed care's implicit minimization of the "other than medical necessity" aspects of a person's life.

Remaining aware of all these intricacies is a formidable task. This is especially true when reality impinges upon and interferes with the patient's and/or the therapist's most vulnerable conflicts. This happens, for example, when the managed care entity is considered to be responding capriciously, rigidly, or unfairly. One doesn't have to look hard in life to uncover a sense of interpersonal unfairness that can readily provoke negative authoritarian transferences—managed care almost calls out for such transference reactions. Yet, even if the managed care entity is benign, its mere existence can foster further complexities. The extent to which these complexities affect the treatment will be determined by many factors, including the patient's level of functioning and the therapist's ability to ascertain and address their impact on the patient and on him/herself. For this reason alone, the effectiveness of a managed care treatment can never be ideal, for there is no room to remain singularly focused on the treatment process without simultaneously attending to the various intrusions of managed care. (For a collection of salient edited essays on the clinical implications of managed care on psychodynamic treatment, see Barron & Sands, 1996.)

The goal of managed care—to keep costs down—means that a managed care system may be potentially detrimental to individual patients. Therefore, each of us must make finer choices: Are there certain companies whose management is not acceptable? Are there certain companies whose management of certain diagnoses is not acceptable? To what extent can we impact and change the way certain companies manage treatment? To what extent can each of us compromise? A couple of examples follow that highlight these issues:

> Company A recruited one of the authors (a psychologist) to be a preferred provider due to a dearth of panel providers in the area who worked with children. A year later, the author was referred an adolescent patient who was being discharged from a partial hospital setting. Briefly, the patient had been hospital-

ized twice for suicidal gestures, had functioned poorly in most spheres of his life for the previous 2 years, and remained very depressed when entering outpatient therapy. After 1 month of twice-weekly treatment and then 10 months of once-a-week treatment, the managed care reviewer communicated to the therapist that for any more sessions to be authorized the patient had to have a psychiatric consultation. The consultation took place and the recommendation from the psychiatrist (one supplied by Company A) was to continue with the treatment plan that the therapist was following. A few more sessions were authorized. Then the author was written a letter stating that in 60 days he would no longer be considered a participating provider for Company A. Given the author's numerous dealings with Company A, which left him believing that there was little hope of working in good faith anymore with this organization, he accepted being dropped from the panel and made arrangements with his patient to continue treatment without the managed care company's involvement and at a considerably reduced fee. (In other instances of providers being dropped from a panel, particularly in those states with laws prohibiting no-cause termination and guaranteeing an appeals process [e.g., New York], the provider might be best advised to contest the managed care organization's action for the good of his/her patients.)

While much is omitted here about the way the author (and the patient) experienced working with Company A, ethical and theoretical questions abound in this example. The case is illustrative of our position that some companies' practices may be too rigid or capricious to work with in good enough faith, and that therapists may have to make difficult decisions in order to preserve the integrity of treatment. But how can we be sure of the impact on the patient of "having to submit" to a psychiatric consultation, despite the patient's oft-repeated statements that he would not take medication? Also, what about the impact of transitioning to paying out of pocket. Certainly the therapist tried to track the manifest and latent derivatives of these events (and other intrusions by working with the reviewer) and address them as they arose, yet how can one ever be certain of doing so sufficiently, especially when the therapist is aware of his own intense reactions to the managed care company? On the other hand, the therapist in this case believes that the patient did make great improvement in many spheres of his life. For example, after having failed 11th grade 2 years in a row, he not only eventually graduated but also became very involved in extracurricular activities. He made more friends, got along better with his parents, secured and kept a part-time job, and severely reduced his use of substances. At the close of treatment, he manifested much greater self-esteem and self-confidence, and he no longer was vexed by his self-injurious impulses. In sum, this was a very successful, though not ideal, psychotherapeutic endeavor.

This next example is provided to suggest that sometimes a company's management philosophy and/or practice may be off-putting, but still avoids the disruption of treatment needs, or at least some treatment needs:

> The patient was referred by one of her friends at work. In the initial consultation the therapist learned that the patient had coverage managed by Company B. (Company B's protocol is to authorize one or two sessions before requiring that a treatment report be submitted for further sessions.) The patient made clear that she had to use her benefits due to her financial situation. Thus, the therapist knew that he needed to make an assessment of her needs based on the potential resources provided by Company B. The therapist and the patient agreed on the following: Her primary reason for presenting for psychotherapy had to do specifically with her difficulties performing at work, especially in regards to her numerous absences and "sick" days. This self-defeating behavior was a reenactment of many disappointing experiences in which her dependency needs went ignored. She had experienced much neglect by both parents, and had often been emotionally forgotten in the midst of her brother's chronic suicidality, her mother's alcoholism, and her father's abandonment of the family. Further, she had spent many years herself in an alcoholic "fog" prior to achieving sobriety without any outside support from family, friends, or treatment. Her present difficulty was conceptualized as reflecting a desire to have someone else take responsibility for her; for example, making sure she got up for work, despite her wish to stay home and be taken care of. A number of times in the initial consultation, the patient evidenced transferential manifestations of her unmet dependency wishes, and

these were commented on by the therapist. The therapist also commented on how, under certain circumstances, they could together potentially allow these wishes to emerge more freely in the therapeutic relationship, but that to do so productively would necessitate meeting more frequently than Company B would probably authorize. (The therapist had arrived at this belief due to his prior experience with Company B, including having attended a meeting in which the company delineated its authorization policies, in addition to his having spoken a number of times with the director about authorization criteria. The therapist was certain that the company would not support any treatment that fostered a benign regression.)

As the therapy unfolded, the therapist experienced some consternation in not attending more openly to his patient's character needs and, further, experienced some interpersonal pressure from the patient that contradicted their agreement to focus the treatment mainly on helping her not miss any further work. Nonetheless, the treatment was quite successful vis-à-vis the agreed-upon goals. After a couple of months, the patient reported that she was no longer on probation at work and that, indeed, she had received a favorable evaluation. The patient also appeared more pleased with herself than previously, though there still was evidence of her being disappointed that more change in her affective experience had not been accomplished.

In this case, did the therapist do what was best for the patient? Was the patient's better functioning in the occupational realm in itself beneficial enough, given that it entailed mitigating and failing to reexplore the emerging dependent transference, as well as foregoing character work that might have been transformative for her? While the patient's short-term and long-term needs bespoke similar underlying dynamics, the former invited an ego-supportive approach and the latter a potentially more profound and developmentally robust transference neurosis. Is it good enough that the patient chose the ego-supportive approach based on her resources (financial and time investment), as well as her decision to focus on changing her behavior over changing her experience of self in relation to the world? Though these remain open questions, there are certain guidelines which we do advocate, such as remaining available to the patient for as long as the patient decides to remain in treatment.

We subscribe to the practice that when we accept patients in the unusual triad of managed care, we accept them to the extent that we will continue our work as long as it is indicated, no matter how the management of the therapy unfolds (providing that we do so within the parameters of our legal/contractual obligations to the managed care company, and providing that these parameters don't undermine our ethical obligations to patients). This means that a number of variables will have to be considered by the therapist if the managed care company denies further authorization (we must remember that this is a financial issue on the manifest level but likely carries all sorts of meanings—for the patient and for the therapist—on the latent level). To break this down further, the notion of additional treatment being "indicated" needs more delineation.

Whether we like it or not, this position entails that *there may be times when we believe that managed care's denial of further authorization is contrary to our belief concerning what the patient needs and in conflict with our legal/ethical obligation, and that now it is up to us to rectify this situation so that the patient can have the opportunity to do the work that is necessary.* This involves the reality-based issues of fee, scheduling, and acceptance of the open-ended nature of working through. It also involves all of the transference and countertransference implications of being the therapist who responds to the patient's needs (i.e., "They [managed care] do not see the importance of continuing this journey, but I do"). Finally, it implies that situations may develop wherein the denial of managed care authorization interacts with the patient's conflicts in such a way that there is no good outcome. These are risks we are taking, and sometimes they do not work out. For example, a patient was seen in once-a-week treatment for a year and a half. At that point, a new policy was initiated by the payer of services that psychotherapy could not last longer than 1 year. This resulted in the prospect that individual treatment would have to be terminated; if the patient wanted further psychotherapy, he would have to accept a referral to a group format. The patient was so unsettled by this unexpected change that he was unable to enter into a self-pay arrangement just between himself and the therapist. A precipitous termination ensued; the therapist was not able to make contact with the patient again, even by telephone. Such endings are unfortunate, at times tragic, and leave the therapist (and the patient also) with many questions that may never be answered.

The inclusion of managed care in the treatment dyad implies that there will be experiences with patients that cannot be understood to the extent we desire and hope for. Yet, we have never lived in a culture that, for the most part, values what psychodynamic psychotherapists value in terms of making sense and meaning out of the interpersonal matrix. Indeed, if there were such a culture, it would need far fewer psychotherapists.

2

Charting New Territory

Psychotherapy is a profession and a business—these two functions are indivisible. While it has been anathema to many clinicians, especially psychodynamic clinicians, to focus on the business side of the practice, the current health care marketplace makes such a focus essential. This is not optimal for the field, but it is the prevailing trend at the moment. How best to respond to this trend is a question with serious implications for both personal fulfillment and financial stability, not to mention clinical integrity. It is a question that each clinician must resolve for him/herself. In the previous chapter we presented many of the clinical implications of working with the managed care triad and considered how these implications resonate with each therapist's determination of whether or not to work with managed care for a particular patient. We don't try to hide our opinion on this question, as we have already articulated. *Simply stated, we encourage much fuller knowledge of managed care by psychodynamic clinicians and a consideration of working within its parameters when that makes sense for one's practice and patients, as well as the ability to advocate against it when that makes most sense. Our intent is not to convince you of any particular stance. Rather, it is to acknowledge the obvious realities and examine a range of possible responses.* In order to do this, we use this second chapter to answer questions such as the following: What is the structure of the managed care world?

How can a psychodynamic clinician engage with it? What are the implications for confidentiality of doing so?

From a business perspective, there are few psychodynamic clinicians for whom managed care has not affected their practice. Whether you have chosen to work directly with it or not, for most independent practitioners it has diminished the volume of self-pay referrals, limited insurance reimbursement levels, and, if you are working with managed care, increased dramatically the amount of time spent doing paperwork. On the other hand, some clinicians have joined provider panels wherein they are directly referred a relatively high volume of patients from the managed care organization, and some clinicians (although less so psychodynamically oriented ones) have secured jobs within managed care organizations. For example, one psychologist with a general psychodynamic practice in a large U.S. east coast city who has contracted with several managed care organizations as a network provider reports: "Six to eight years ago most of my referrals came from other colleagues or by word of mouth. Now about two-thirds come from managed care organizations. Even though all the extra paperwork is burdensome, I do have a steadier stream of referrals, for now."

APPROACHES TO MANAGED CARE

There are three fundamental stances that we see psychodynamic clinicians adopting regarding managed care:

The first is characterized by both assimilation and accommodation, in which the clinician assimilates the goals and accommodates to the practices of psychotherapy in a managed care environment. In doing so, he/she might work within a health maintenance organization (HMO) or provider partnership (to be discussed below) dedicated to brief treatment and focused on acute symptom reduction, or might work in an administrative role in a managed care organization or acute hospital setting.

The second stance is characterized by accommodation to managed care practices without full assimilation of the goals of managed care. Within this stance a clinician would try to maintain a traditional outpatient psychotherapy practice with some self-pay patients, when the referrals present on their own, but simultaneously contract with managed care organizations to become an affiliated provider of problem-focused treatment of patients obtained through the organization's referral structure.

The third stance is characterized by rejection of the goals and practices of managed care, in an attempt to maintain an outpatient practice without any managed care intrusion (which increasingly means foregoing any third-party reimbursement, as fewer conventional nonmanaged major medical plans still exist). Often paramount for those adopting this stance is an understandable repudiation of the transcending of boundaries around confidentiality that working with managed care necessitates, as well as rejecting third-party-imposed limitations on the duration of treatment. For others adopting this stance, the decision is a financial one, wherein their self-pay referral base is strong enough that they calculate sufficient referrals without network participation. Additionally, as managed care organizations have increasingly limited reimbursement levels and require much nonreimbursed paperwork time, carrying on a practice even with reduced fees relative to managed care may make more financial sense.

Not many psychodynamic clinicians are adopting the first stance of assimilation and accommodation. This is because it implies a complete embrace of a managed care treatment-limiting approach to virtually all presenting problems, and such an approach is not consistent with a general psychodynamic practice in which some patients will need intermediate to long-term psychotherapy, not to mention the myriad other ethical and technical constraints of managed care. The remainder (and majority) of psychodynamic clinicians seem divided between the second stance of accommodation and the third stance of rejection.

POLITICS AND STRUCTURE
OF MANAGED CARE

Managed care, or at least some incarnation of cost control measures, is an inevitable outgrowth of a health care system that was increasingly out of control fiscally. Throughout the 1980s there were unending reports of spiraling health care costs which outstripped inflation

by many times. Although mental health providers, and psychodynamics practitioners in particular, were not the real culprits
here, we are part of a larger health care system that had become
increasingly costly and relatively unregulated. That we, along
with other health service providers, could receive third-party reimbursement by submitting therapy bills with no other documentation came to be the standard of our business practice. In
fact, it helped promote the illusion that we weren't really engaged in a business (which we are), but merely providers of a
professional and human service (which we still are).

Given the need for fiscal restraint and "reengineering" following the Reagan era swell of corporate and governmental
spending and the ballooning of the federal deficit, the health
care system was a natural target. It accounts for a major portion
of the gross domestic product, and it had been largely unregulated from a fiscal perspective. If we in the mental health field
had been clairvoyant and initiated regulatory and cost-cutting
steps from within (an admittedly difficult thing to do), we might
have held off the surge of managed care, but not necessarily.
Managed care is a reification of a cultural/economic trend that
reaches much further than the health care system and does not
in its current incarnation reflect the end stage of evolution. We
expect that it will continue to evolve, as the national trend of trying to wring more out of less (i.e., increase earnings growth
faster than revenue growth) continues. This trend may have been
inevitable, but it is at present difficult to adjust to. Just as most
people seem to be working harder over the past few years to
maintain the same level of income, psychotherapists, especially
those working with third-party payers, are having to spend 20–
30% more time documenting and communicating about the
work they are doing for 20–30% less in reimbursement. To maintain income at present levels, the solution for many has been to
see more patients—not an easy route. Others have maintained
current practice levels and grudgingly accepted a lower income—
also not a favorable outcome. Some have left the clinical domain
entirely, opting instead for administrative roles or retirement.

Considering the current ubiquity of the term "managed
care," it is amazing to think that 15 years ago barely anyone had
heard of it. It has evolved over a relatively short period of time to

connote a financially driven management template that is applied to the health care system. Yet, within this template are numerous concepts and procedures, each relevant to particular constituencies within health care, whether it be consumers, insurance companies, clinicians, human resource managers, or quality control reviewers. For the purposes of this book, we are most interested in those concepts relevant to the ways in which mental health clinicians function in a managed care environment: HMO, EAP, PPO, traditional indemnity, and IPA. As these terms are central to the health care marketplace, we review them each briefly below for those clinicians for whom they are not yet clear.

HMOs (health maintenance organizations) were the first incarnation of managed care in the health field. In an HMO, mental health clinicians usually function on a salaried basis. They treat only patients who are members of that HMO and who have been referred by their primary care physician, acting as a gatekeeper for specialized services. Occasionally, HMOs will contract with adjunct providers to offer services not fully staffed in-house. In an HMO there may or may not be a predetermined limit to the number of sessions permissible, but even if no limit exists there is reinforcement for limiting the utilization of services.

The prospect for a psychodynamic clinician securing a job in an HMO depends in part on training and in part on orientation to treatment. Aside from the need for a few MDs who have a largely gatekeeper and medicating function, less training may in fact be more marketable in an HMO context. Since the function of a mental health clinician is usually very brief treatment and crisis intervention, high levels of training are often deemed less necessary and more expensive. Therefore, this venue may provide good opportunities for the nonspecific master's level clinician or psychiatric social worker. A psychodynamic approach to treatment does not preclude working in an HMO setting as long as you are well versed in and comfortable practicing short-term dynamic psychotherapy, as well as utilizing other modalities when needed. This mix of expertise and affinities is not something to which most dynamic clinicians will ascribe; for those that do fit this mix, working in an HMO can provide a stable income at the cost of less depth treatment and a very large case-load.

EAPs (employee assistance plans) have become more common in recent years in large corporate and organizational settings. An EAP (for mental health and substance abuse) typically consists of one or more providers, either on salary or on a contractual basis, that act as a first-line resource for employees experiencing mental health difficulties. There is typically a maximum number of visits allowed with an EAP clinician (usually between 2 and 10), and if further treatment is needed the clinician then refers the employee outside of the organization for further treatment. An EAP is not designed to offer a full range or a long-term treatment option, but rather to function as an acute care resource and triage mechanism for employees in need.

The potential role of a psychodynamic clinician in an EAP is not dissimilar to that within an HMO. One must be familiar with and willing to deliver primarily short-term interventions, and also must be at least somewhat fluent in other treatment modalities. Since an EAP intervention is by definition short term and aimed at triage, many EAP patients are referred out for longer-term therapy.

A *PPO* (preferred provider organization) refers to a panel of clinicians that has been selected by the managed care organization and/or insurance company to provide services to any patients seeking them out, or referred to them, who are insured by that company. Provider fees are usually set on a contractual basis at a fixed rate for a given type of service within a given geographic region (e.g., a managed care organization may reimburse $75 for a 45-minute psychotherapy session in the San Francisco area, while the same service may garner only $60 in the California state capital area of Sacramento). A clinician treating a patient through a PPO usually has to gain ongoing authorization for continued treatment from a managed care reviewer or primary care physician, and there may be a maximum number of yearly visits permissible or yearly dollar cap. (A variant of a PPO plan is a point of service [POS] plan, which essentially offers PPO-like provider options for little copayment from the patient, as well as the opportunity to see any nonpanel provider for a somewhat greater cost to the patient.)

PPO panels represent one of the best points of entry in the managed care world for psychodynamic clinicians. This is because the large numbers of providers on each panel allow them to support a more diverse range of specialties and orientations than does an HMO or EAP, which typically have a limited number of clinicians on staff. As well, a clinician does not have to work exclusively with a particular panel, allowing for a mixed practice of one or more PPO and other self-pay patients. We know scores of psychodynamically oriented clinicians whose practices function, in part, with patients who are insured under PPOs. These clinicians then can develop a balance of short- and long-term treatments, supportive and insight oriented. There is, however, one formidable catch for a member of a PPO panel: if your average treatment length for patients on that panel are high over time, you will likely find yourself getting far fewer referrals from that managed care organization. While such a policy of "nonpreferred" preferred providers is not generally publicized, experiential data suggest that it is standard practice for many managed care organizations.

To become part of a PPO panel, clinicians must usually submit an extensive application and sign a contract that stipulates the nature of the relationship with the insurance company and the patient. These applications often contain some rather unpalatable stipulations in the areas of confidentiality, conditions for termination of the contract, and—more uncommonly—indemnity against appeals or litigation against the managed care organization. Before signing any contract, a clinician would be well advised to *read it carefully,* as it will likely contain many contentious points whose implications need to be understood completely. For those who find all of these challenges of the application process impossible to live with, working with a PPO is obviously not an option. For those psychodynamic clinicians who are willing to work within these parameters, it can be a productive relationship. What is important when trying to gain inclusion into a network is presenting a unique set of skills and expertise, and fashioning a cover letter that uses the appropriate language to describe one's psychodynamic orientation and interventions. Such descriptors as *psychoanalytic, transference-based, interpretive,* and *insight-oriented* are red flags that can scare off the managed care organization. Alternative and roughly similar descriptors such as, respectively, *interpersonal, relationship history, cognitive reappraisal,* and *promoting reality testing* would be more understandable to someone reviewing your application. (There is more on this linguistic issue in Chapter Four, and for pragmatic information on applying to a PPO, there are several useful references cited in Appendix A.)

The notion of *traditional indemnity* refers to the way insurance companies, through major medical plans, have reimbursed any licensed providers for offering clinical services in their offices. In other words, a patient desiring psychotherapy has the option of seeking out any willing and licensed provider, and is usually subject to yearly or lifetime maximums on number of sessions or payments available. In traditional indemnity plans, there is typically no managed care review of services. While traditional indemnity plans are being offered less and less frequently by insurance companies, there is a growing consumer, legislative, and clinician movement to mandate a traditional indemnity option in all insurance plans, albeit at somewhat reduced reimbursement rates and with higher insurance premiums, than when utilizing clinicians within a PPO panel.

For the psychodynamic clinician, the traditional indemnity plan may at first seem the obvious plan of choice, but this needs to be critically evaluated. The situation 15 and more years ago was certainly appealing, when traditional indemnity plans had high per session and per year limits and often paid 80% of most submitted session fees. Current traditional indemnity plans, and those likely to develop in the near future, are not nearly so generous. The per year maximum dollar amounts are rather restrictive, and in fact there are often higher yearly levels available under PPO plans. The great draw for a clinician of any orientation to traditional indemnity plans is that there is no management of the care offered by a third-party reviewer and there is far less paperwork demanded.

Finally, *IPA* (independent practice association), or group practice, a more recent provider configuration in the mental health field, refers to a group of independent clinicians who form a partnership that collectively negotiates with health insurance companies and/or managed care organizations to treat patients covered under a particular insurance plan. Clinicians within IPAs usually represent the spectrum of mental health disciplines. An IPA can be characterized as functioning like a small-scale HMO for mental health problems. One possible characteristic of an IPA's contract with an insurance company is a *capitation provision,* which means that rather than the company reimbursing the IPA separately for each patient visit, the company and the IPA negotiate a set fee for each covered life (i.e., each insured person within a given geographic or employer group who can potentially seek out services). The advantage to capitation for both the insurance company and the IPA is that costs/income are fixed, guaranteed, and paid in advance; the potential disadvantage for the IPA is that if the provider group underestimates the potential utilization of services it may be caught in a situation where it doesn't have adequate provider resources for the number of presenting patients yet still remain contractually obligated to provide these services.

There may be much appeal to an IPA for a psychodynamic clinician, as the provider group sets internal standards for treatment review and quality (notwithstanding certain omnibus standards imposed by insurers, licensing bodies, and professional organizations). Thus, an IPA can (potentially) readily support psychodynamic practice, as long as it is practiced in a form that isn't always depth treatment. The ethical dilemma for the IPA is that if a considerable number of patients are offered long-term, insight-oriented treatment, there is no additional payment for this, as fees are contracted for on a per capita rather than services-rendered basis. Still, given the relative control that an IPA has in establishing its own mix of providers and modalities, it may be quite attractive for a psychodynamic practitioner.

CONFIDENTIALITY AND PROTECTION OF THE PATIENT–THERAPIST RELATIONSHIP

One of the primary and most distressing concerns of psychodynamic clinicians regarding managed care is the issue of the confidentiality (or lack thereof) of clinical information and the potential impact third-party reimbursement may have on a psychotherapeutic relationship. This is a serious issue, and one that will affect certain treatments more than others. Managed care organizations would argue that third-party reimbursement is not a mandatory enterprise and that if an individual is contracting with a company for health care payments, he/she needs to abide by that company's rules for exchange of information. From the clinician's perspective, exchange of information involves, at best, a breach of therapist–patient confidentiality and, at worst, a threat to the therapeutic alliance and possibly the treatment outcome. A clinical social worker, trained as an analyst, expressed these concerns this way: "I haven't had a lot to do with managed care—anything that curtails a psychotherapist's freedom is a scary thing. Any intrusion into the therapeutic relationship complicates what is already a sensitive situation. It's a burden that has to be thought through by the therapist and that will undoubtedly have an impact on the patient."

Working with managed care organizations does present the clinician with an ethical dilemma (Small & Barnhill, 1998). Psychotherapists are bound by the rules of privileged communication, except in the case of clear and present danger to the patient, threat by the patient toward another person, report or clear intent of engaging in abuse toward a minor, or when a specific release of information has been executed. This latter circumstance is a must before any therapist shares information with managed care reviewers. Having the patient read and sign a release of information regarding sharing of clinical and historical information with the managed care organization "covers" you legally, but the problem remains that confidentiality has come to be an expectable (and theoretically congruent) aspect of psychodynamic psychotherapy, and breaching it is not an ideal option under any circumstance.

While we agree with the fundamental premise that an enduring therapeutic alliance is a key element of successful psychodynamic psychotherapy, we do not agree that the appropriate sharing of information with a managed care organization necessarily destroys this alliance. Our data for this assertion are from experiential as well as from anecdotal reports we hear from colleagues who work with managed care. What seems to be a pivotal factor for these therapists with relative success in maintaining a working alliance is the institution of a treatment frame which, from the beginning, makes clear to the patient the necessity of sharing information and addresses quite explicitly what type of information will be shared. Also useful is a reminder to the patient that, as with any presentation of information, one has to make choices about what is presented. Both the clinician and patient therefore have roles in deciding what to share. Finally, patients need to know that a choice is available to not share information, although this means the likely reduction or foregoing of third-party reimbursement. Having taken these steps initially with the patient regarding confidentiality, should his/her concerns or fantasies regarding this issue later arise, they can more readily be explored and worked through therapeutically.

There is a range of treatments for which a breach of confidentiality can pose a real threat to the alliance, such as in insight-oriented therapy with borderline spectrum patients, supportive or insight-oriented therapy with paranoid patients, or any insight-oriented treatment where there are strong and dominating transference paradigms regularly enacted by the patient. In such cases, the most ethical treatment decision may be to forego third-party reimbursement, or accept the lower "out-of-network provider" non-managed care reimbursement level, in favor of an unobstructed treatment where no third party is involved. But what about a patient who can't begin to afford treatment without third-party reimbursement? This too poses a tough ethical question which forces the clinician to balance nonoptimal factors. We believe that effectively and ethically balancing these factors represents one of the greatest challenges to a psychodynamic psychotherapist's decision about whether to work with managed care or not.

3

Treatment Authorization
Opportunities and Dilemmas

In the first two chapters we discussed the structure and dynamics of the managed care world as they pertain to psychodynamic psychotherapists. We now turn attention to the more process-oriented issue of gaining treatment authorization. This refers to the gatekeeping function of managed care, which is really its main calling or raison d'être in the "management" of treatment provision. In this chapter, we provide some background information about who the treatment reviewers are and what they are looking for, as well as suggestions on gaining authorization for patients with differing intrapsychic and functional clusters.

THE NOTION OF MEDICAL NECESSITY

The fundamental goals of clinicians and health insurers are not entirely dissimilar, although they have diametrically opposing emphases: psychodynamic clinicians attempt to provide a meaningful human service and to make money, whereas health insurers attempt to make money and provide a needed human service. The significant differential is in the relative motivation toward making money versus providing a human service, and the means one takes to achieve these goals. For managed care, making money is clearly *the* goal. When approached from this perspective, what becomes important to remember in negotiating with the managed care gatekeepers is that "unnecessary" expenditures make them nervous. What is of paramount importance for a clinician who decides to work with managed care is assuring the organization that the service provided is of "medical necessity." This includes the notions of (1) *treatment need* (i.e., the patient presents a diagnosis and symptom picture that are reasonably treatable), (2) *clinical efficacy* (i.e., a given treatment has demonstrated results), and (3) *cost efficacy* (i.e., a given treatment is less costly in comparison to other equivalent treatments). The first issue, that of treatment need, is one which most psychodynamic clinicians are reasonably well equipped to address and is also the subject of much recent discussion and writings. It involves presenting a managed care reviewer with a diagnostic profile and current symptom picture which indicate that the need for treatment is real and present, and emphasize that if such treatment were not undertaken, further and more expensive problems and treatments would likely ensue. (The specific language and structure of communications about treatment need will be addressed in the next two chapters.) The rationales of clinical and of cost efficacy are ones that have some clear and documentable support in the outcomes and assessment literatures, but are not as readily known or available to most clinicians, and will be taken up in Chapter Seven.

Medical necessity has been the gold standard of the health care industry for a long time, and with the advent of managed care has reached the mental health domain full force. It is a lamentable but current reality that psychotherapies aimed at promoting a fuller and more fulfilling life in an otherwise functionally intact individual are no longer valued by the health insurance industry. In fact, such therapies may never have been valued, but they were reimbursed out of historical disinterest in the micromanagement of treatment provision—as long as a patient had a DSM axis I (and sometimes axis II) diagnosis, treatment was reimbursed. Circumstances have changed dramatically in a brief period of time. Medical necessity is now approached by various managed care organizations from slightly different perspectives, but typically it incorporates the general notions of treatment need, clinical efficacy, and cost efficacy outlined above.

WHO ARE THE TREATMENT REVIEWERS AND HOW DO I COMMUNICATE WITH THEM?

A point of profound frustration for many psychotherapists trying to gain treatment authorization concerns the professional qualifications of the managed care organization's treatment reviewers. The first level of a case's review, either in written or verbal form, is usually done by individuals with little or no formal training in mental health. They commonly have bachelor's or master's level degrees and have been trained by the managed care organization in treatment protocols and quality-review criteria. The absence of treatment experience and professional training among this first level of reviewers is disturbing. We have heard so often of clinicians feeling offended that paraprofessionals are evaluating the treatments offered by fully trained professionals. We concur with this attitude. Managed care organizations should have only professionally trained reviewers evaluating treatments, which in some cases they do (usually nurses or master's level professionals). This level of training should become the standard for all first-level review. For the next level of review, which involves complicated cases, those needing treatment for long periods, or appeals on initial reviews, there are usually professionally trained individuals at the RN, MSW, MD, or PhD level doing the work. Perhaps the only bright spot, of sorts, in the initial treatment review process is that we suspect that many written requests for recertification are barely read, or not read at all. Thus, with many organizations the treatment report becomes merely a gatekeeping and documentation tool, rather than a clinical tool.

Notwithstanding the serious concerns about reviewers' professional qualifications, our experience has been that most reviewers act with relative reason and in accordance with their company's internal (and sometimes externally disseminated) guidelines for treatment review. There are certainly apocryphal stories about misinformed decisions on the part of treatment reviewers, and we too have experienced a few. There may also be a tendency on the part of some clinicians to engage in overattribution of expertise, authority, and/or hostility concerning these reviewers. Beyond anything, they are usually just people trying to do a job for which they were trained, and they respond best when treated with decency and politeness. Condescending or ingratiating attitudes on the part of clinicians go a long way toward souring the relationship, and there *is* a relationship. This point would seem so obvious as to be unnecessary to state explicitly, but it is so often violated that it bears emphasizing. Legitimate disagreements with either the substance or rules governing authorization decisions are best taken up with supervisors or senior clinicians/reviewers.

Still, one of the hardest things to stomach about the managed care review process is that there is a third party involved in making treatment decisions regarding you and your patients and, while not usually capricious, these decisions are sometimes unpalatable. We have no interest in trying to rationalize this aspect of managed care—it is one of the distasteful elements that each clinician has to consider in deciding whether to work within this system or not.

SECURING TREATMENT AUTHORIZATION AND THIRD-PARTY REIMBURSEMENT

As we approach the fiscal realities of the health insurance system in the coming years, we need to be savvy in our use of managed care. We must know how to obtain third-party reimbursement when it is available to and appropriate for a particular patient, and seek other sources of reimbursement when a patient seeks a treatment which we know won't be authorized.

In evaluating the likelihood of reimbursement of a given psychodynamic treatment, it may be useful to think of two intersecting dimensions: functional impairment and intrapsychic impairment. Functional impairment refers to the level at which a patient can adaptively engage in regular work, sustain meaningful interpersonal relationships, and live independently, and the extent to which psychological distress and symptom formation impair such functioning. Intrapsychic impairment refers to the level of ego resources, adaptive defenses, appropriate superego controls and sublimatory channels, and the interaction of these factors in producing or diminishing psychological conflict and distress. The interaction of these two dimensions results in four quadrants: functional impairment–intrapsychic impairment; functional impairment–intrapsychic adaptation; functional adaptation–intrapsychic impairment; and functional adaptation–intrapsychic adaptation. This four quadrant model can be useful in evaluating both the likelihood of managed care reimbursement and the question of which form of psychodynamic treatment to pursue, and is represented graphically in Figure 1. (In discussing which form of treatment to pursue, we suggest largely psychodynamic treatments, yet recognize that other modalities of treatment are often equally or more indicated.)

Functional Impairment–Intrapsychic Impairment

This is the quadrant wherein managed care treatment authorization and reimbursement are most likely to occur, given that impairment exists in functioning, which is the overarching bench-

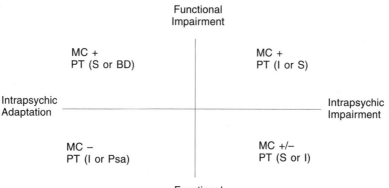

FIGURE 1. Managed care reimbursement likelihood and psychotherapeutic indicators. MC, managed care reimbursement likelihood (+ or –); PT, psychotherapy (S, supportive; I, insight-oriented; BD, brief dynamic; Psa, psychoanalysis). *Note.* This figure represents the likelihood of managed care reimbursement for various forms of psychodynamic treatment under differing functional and intrapsychic conditions. It does not include other models of therapy, many of which may also be applicable to the quadrants above.

mark, as well as intrapsychically. A patient in this quadrant might, for example, be clinically depressed and having a hard time getting up each morning for work, experiencing marital conflict, feeling very angry at a coworker but unable to express it constructively, and overwhelmed with guilt at not having been available enough as a father, just as he felt his parents were not available for him. Such a patient would likely be authorized for treatment of a moderate to relatively long-term duration. He complains of multiple functional impairments associated with depression, marital, and work stressors, as well as a potentially complicated guilt reaction. The presence of the latter intrapsychic distress, coexisting with what may be an introjective depression, presents evidence that he might make good use of a supportive or insight-oriented psychodynamic psychotherapy following initial relief of the marked depressive symptoms.

Functional Impairment–Intrapsychic Adaptation

This quadrant represents one in which a managed care organization would be likely to authorize treatment given the level of functional impairment, but where a psychodynamic psychotherapy may be less indicated than a behavioral therapy given the underlying level of intrapsychic (i.e., character) adaptation. When a psychodynamic psychotherapy could be useful, it would likely be either a supportive treatment that addresses behavioral functioning in a pragmatic, albeit psychodynamic, fashion or a brief dynamic therapy that revolves around a clear problem focus. A patient falling within this quadrant might be exemplified by a woman experiencing procrastination difficulties on work projects, which are putting her job status in jeopardy. Treatment for this focal problem is likely to be short term. A critical question in determining which form of brief treatment to pursue is the extent to which the maladaptive behavior can be ameliorated through improved scheduling, work habits, etc., arguing for a behavioral approach, or whether it is symptomatic of an internally conflictual stressor, for which a psychodynamic approach could be useful. If the stressor is eliciting a focal developmental conflict (i.e., Oedipal guilt), then a brief dynamic therapy might be indicated; if the stressor is the primary issue without underlying developmental conflict, then a supportive therapy would likely be indicated.

Functional Adaptation–Intrapsychic Impairment

The likelihood of managed care authorization for treatment of a patient within this quadrant is uncertain. Level of functioning is the strongest benchmark when a managed care organization evaluates the need for treatment, but if significant intrapsychic conflict and nonbehaviorally enacted emotional distress are present, it may be authorized. Such a case might be represented by a college student who is able to perform well in classes, structure her time appropriately, and engage in a reasonably intimate relationship, but experiences enormous ambivalence and felt distress about making broad choices in her life, such as which career direction to pursue and whether to become engaged to her boyfriend. For this patient, functional level traditionally has been and continues to be adaptive, yet internally there is significant conflict and distress precipitated by increasing developmental tasks. While the need for psychotherapy to ensure basic functioning is minimal in managed care terms, the patient could most likely benefit from a brief- to moderate-duration therapy of a supportive or insight-oriented nature. Whether such treatment would be authorized might hinge on the extent to which, without current intervention, the intrapsychic impairment would be likely to produce functional impairment requiring a more intensive level of care in the near future, as well as any history of similar conflicts leading to functional impairment.

Functional Adaptation–Intrapsychic Adaptation

This quadrant represents the one least likely to qualify for third-party reimbursement under a managed care system, wherein a patient is functionally and intrapsychically operating at adaptive levels yet seeks treatment in order to enhance self-awareness and/or to further improve character functioning and quality of life. In this case an insight-oriented therapy or psychoanalysis might be of much use and clinically indicated, but not of any functional or intrapsychic medical necessity, which is the managed care litmus test.

As should be clear from this discussion of levels of functional and intrapsychic impairment/adaptation, a clinician's judgment that psychodynamic treatment could be useful is not identical with a managed care organization's notion of medical necessity. In some of the quadrants there is much overlap of these two perspectives, but particularly in the last one discussed there is little overlap. The importance of understanding areas of convergence and divergence of clinician and managed care organization perspectives is that *the style in which a clinician conceptualizes and writes up a treatment request for a managed care organization is vitally important to gaining authorization.* By style we mean (1) clarity and generalizability of the clinical language used, (2) recognition of the notion of differing treatment necessities, and (3) demonstration of active critical decision making regarding treatment necessity. While not all clinically useful psychodynamic psychotherapies will be authorized under a managed care system, many will *if* the clinician presents the case appropriately to the task. This conditionality to authorization is most relevant for the functional adaptation–intrapsychic impairment quadrant, where the presence of current good functioning challenges the clinician to effectively document the nuances of the need for treatment on intrapsychic grounds.

CONTINUED PSYCHOTHERAPY AFTER MANAGED CARE AUTHORIZATION ENDS

After a psychotherapist has gained authorization for treatment from a managed care organization, yet another problematic situation may arise, which we began to describe clinically in earlier chapters. This involves cases where continued treatment is indicated and either the managed care reviewer disagrees or the patient's insurance benefits run out. Of all the thorny issues involved in working with managed care, these two related problems may be the most treacherous.

If you are a provider on a managed care panel (PPO), you should be aware of any contract provision, or lack thereof, regarding continued treatment after authorization ends. There is no rule that applies to all organizations, although many companies do specify that you abide by their authorization decisions. Let's begin by considering the simplest of situations. Assume you have been treating a 23-year-old dysthymic patient with a dependent character disorder for an initial 10-session authorization, beginning in March, which the managed care organization automatically granted upon the patient's request for treatment. You then completed an OTR (outpatient treatment report) and requested 15 additional sessions, for which they authorized 12 on a once-per-week basis. You then completed an OTR requesting 8 more sessions, which they approved. These 30 sessions constituted the maximum outpatient psychotherapy benefit available for this patient in any calendar year. Having completed all 30 sessions by October, you find that the patient is less depressed and feeling reasonably productive, but is experiencing considerable distress about his/her inability to sustain a lasting intimate relationship. Continued treatment of at least a moderate duration is indicated to consolidate a working through of the dependency enactments and relational failures, and the patient is willing to self-pay at a somewhat reduced fee. According to your contract with the managed care organization, there are no limitations on treatment following authorization that would contradict your clinical judgment, and the patient's ability to self-pay obviously would justify continued treatment.

Now let's add a complication to this situation. In January, after you have seen the patient for a total of 42 sessions, insurance benefits potentially become available again as it is a new calendar year. In order to receive benefits, you will need to complete further OTRs over time, and the question arises regarding the manner in which you present the clinical work already done to the managed care organization. In this case, you must be clear (i.e., not lie) about the continuing nature of the treatment but simultaneously be able to document the current clinical status as one representing a need for treatment. In other words, be honest about what you have done, but beyond that regard the write-up almost as if it were the first, by arguing for a compelling need for treatment. While there is no guarantee, you are likely to receive continued authorization as long as you can make a strong case that there are active clinical signs and functional impairments being treated, not just that you and the patient don't want to stop therapy for what some might view as "vague" psychodynamic goals.

An even more complicated scenario arises when your contract with a managed care organization stipulates that you must abide by their authorizations and not treat patients in that plan otherwise. In cases such as this, where benefits have run out for the year, the issue surfaces of medical/clinical necessity and potential liability versus a contractual obligation. You are forced here to balance your potential legal and ethical liability with the patient's needs. As a general rule of thumb, don't do anything that puts you at risk of malpractice—if you assess that the patient absolutely needs further treatment, provide it. An intermediary step that can help to indemnify you is to ask a colleague to do a consultation on the patient regarding the need for treatment. This will add weight to your argument for treatment, should the question arise. Another possible step is to document that the managed care organization's recommendation is below the standard of care for the patient's diagnosis, and provide a copy to the patient. In any case, when communicating with the managed care organization for subsequent authorization, you must be clear about the nature and frequency of treatment you have provided, and strongly emphasize the issue of clinical necessity and the risks if treatment were not to be continued. Managed care organizations are very sensitive to liability risks and ballooning costs, so if you present a coherent case that without treatment this patient will have suffered greatly and perhaps been at risk of more expensive treatment options or personal harm, they are predisposed to listen.

The most challenging and potentially harmful of situations are those where continued benefits are potentially available in a calendar year but the managed care organization denies continued authorization. The approach to take here is not dissimilar from that above, where a balance is forged between clinical necessity and contractual obligation. In this case, however, you generally have the right of appeal under most contracts, and by statute in some states. Consultation with a colleague and documentation from the patient about the viability/need for continued treatment can be helpful. Furthermore, demonstrating that additional problems would likely arise should treatment not continue is always called for, when it is in fact true. If, after appeal, treatment is still denied, you have a real dilemma on your hands. We would again suggest erring on the side of solid clinical judgment, even though this stance may risk your inclusion on the managed care panel. Before taking any major steps, an ethical/ legal consultation with your state and/or national professional organization could be useful. Most professional organizations have staff designated for such purposes and are increasingly proactive in supporting legal actions against managed care organizations' "malpractice" of medicine by less than fully trained health care reviewers.

4

Transforming Psychodynamic Concepts into a Managed Care (Functional) Language

When communicating with a managed care reviewer, it is useful to remember that his/her aim is always to understand just enough of the treatment process to be able to authorize just enough therapy as is needed to ensure adaptive functioning, or at least a return to baseline functioning. With this in mind, for most managed care organizations you don't have to tell them much, and what you do tell them should be crisp, concise, functionally based, and clearly indicative of treatment need. The less they have to think and read between the lines, the better. As we noted in Chapter Three when we presented the four-quadrant model, functionality refers to the level at which a patient can adaptively engage in regular work, sustain meaningful interpersonal relationships, and live independently. These activities do not have to be engaged in all at once, only so long as there is the real potential to engage in them.

Psychoanalysis is an intellectual/empirical/clinical theory that guides the practice of psychodynamic psychotherapy. Managed care also has a loose guiding theory, but it is an economic, not an intellectual, one. Both dynamic psychotherapy and managed care have underlying clinical languages. The essential difference is that the clinical language of managed care doesn't follow from its economic theory directly; it borrows from several bodies of clinical theory in the service of describing the treatment situation in ways that support the economic goals of managed care. It draws particularly on those bodies of theory that can be construed as supporting time-limited, and therefore purportedly cost-contained, psychotherapy.

While the language of psychodynamic treatment may seem to be, and often is, at odds with the language of managed care, the interventions are not always at odds. This is the point of departure for this chapter. Notwithstanding the uniqueness of transference-based interventions, many of the other interventions practiced by psychodynamic clinicians are in fact similar to those practiced by psychotherapists working within other modalities, including a managed care framework. Yet the theoretical language of psychodynamic clinicians is not easily understood or valued by managed care companies and is thus viewed with caution or even antipathy.

If you are going to treat managed care patients, you must be aware that the specific form and content of communications with managed care organizations is all-important. As any international traveler knows, people can't readily speak with you if they don't understand your language, and if you do manage somehow to communicate, what you are saying and what they perceive you to be saying may be very different. Misperception doesn't help the cause of getting authorization for your patents.

Having focused in the earlier chapters on the structure of managed care and the clinical indications involved in the treatment authorization process, in this chapter and the next we turn to the specifics of communication with managed care organizations. This chapter in particular addresses those areas of linguistic and theoretical similarity and dissimilarity among psychodynamic psychotherapy and cognitive or behavioral therapies. The task is to take these concepts and use them within a "functional language" in communications, as will be illustrated in the next chapter. The goal here is not to equivocate or to imply that all therapies are essentially similar (which they are not), but instead to demonstrate that there are many techniques that share common roots and that symptoms and treatment effects can be described in an atheoretical language of individual functionality that is not inconsistent with the underlying theory. Such a language is rooted in the principles of mental status examination and the various symptom- and observation-based descriptors that it engages.

Language that is unfamiliar makes treatment reviewers anxious. The same concept put in familiar conceptual and/or functional terms (i.e., those rooted in observable symptoms and daily functioning) can engender a vastly different reception. Some of managed care's wariness about psychodynamics reflects linguistic confusion. You should be able to use the information presented in this chapter to more effectively understand and review the areas of commonality between various theoretical perspectives, and hence to communicate more effectively with managed care companies about patients' functioning. To do so does not mean changing the type of work you do, but rather enhancing your ability to communicate about psychodynamic work in a language that can be widely understood.

We will individually review several fundamental psychodynamic concepts and suggest their cognitive and/or behavioral parallels. These concepts include intrapsychic; transference; therapeutic alliance; working through; defenses (rationalization, projection, suppression, and repression); and interpretation (clarification, confrontation, and interpretation proper). *Whatever the language called for with a given case, we always suggest that instead of describing a treatment to a managed care entity as "psychodynamic," you use the term "interpersonal."* While having a roughly equivalent meaning, the latter term is less loaded for those not well versed in psychodynamics. It is also associated with a body of treatment efficacy research (e.g., the National Institute of Mental Health longitudinal study of depression comparing cognitive-behavioral, interpersonal, and pharmacological treatment paradigms) that enhances its "credibility."

AREAS OF CONCEPTUAL CONVERGENCE

Psychodynamics embodies a complicated and rich set of conceptual principles and therapeutic techniques. Its very complexity is both its draw and its occasional undoing. There is always risk in oversimplifying, and we don't wish to fall into this trap. We do wish to offer suggestions as to specific areas of conceptual overlap between differing theories. The convergences to be discussed reflect a means to communicate in alternative language about psychodynamic work, language that may be more easily understood. Despite some vast differences between these conceptual models in practice, there are nevertheless enough underlying substrates to allow for comparisons.

Table 1 highlights several key psychodynamic concepts and some behavioral and/or cognitive concepts. This is not an exhaustive listing of important psychodynamic concepts. It reflects those for which we believe there is a meaningful comparison in alternative language that can be used to emphasize functionality. At the risk of defending too strenuously against a presumed and understandable critique, we will state just one last time that this is not a list of equivalent concepts, just *parallels* that are worth

TABLE 1. Psychodynamic Concepts and Their Behavioral or Cognitive Parallels

Psychodynamic concept	Behavioral/cognitive/functional concepts
Intrapsychic process	Underlying psychological state
Transference	Cognitive schema; graduated exposure (*in vivo* and imaginal) to earlier relational experience
Therapeutic alliance	Positive attribution; modeling
Working through	Self-efficacy; stimulus control; contingency management; cognitive self-monitoring
Defenses	
Rationalization	Cognitive reconstrual
Projection	External attribution
Suppression	Avoidance
Repression	Exclusion of information
Interpretation	
Clarification	Distancing
Confrontation	Decentering
Interpretation proper	Reattribution; shaping; identifying alternative cognitive patterns

considering when trying to effectively communicate about psychodynamic work.

Below we systematically discuss this list, highlighting the areas of convergence. In doing so, we have drawn upon several useful reference sources on psychodynamic, behavioral, and cognitive concepts (Bongar & Beutler, 1995; Craighead, Craighead, Kazdin, & Mahoney, 1994; Moore & Fine, 1990; Walrond-Skinner, 1986).

The notion of *intrapsychic process* is perhaps the most fundamental concept to psychoanalytic theory and its application in psychodynamic practice. It refers to mental processes that operate within the mind, which in classical psychoanalytic terms means the interaction between the structures of id, ego, and superego operating on three levels—conscious, preconscious, and unconscious. Although this term has come to have such general and common usage in psychology, invoking it actually signifies the psychodynamic belief that much of what occurs mentally is at a level out of awareness, has its own dynamics, and hence internal life. Although the notion of intrapsychic has no actual parallel in alternative language, we thought it important to discuss it and suggest a similar but less psychodynamically oriented term, that of *underlying psychological state*. This description conveys the similar idea of internal mental processes in somewhat more universal language. While the notion of underlying psychological states was antithetical to early work in behavior therapy, more recently both cognitive-behavioral theory and systems theory have integrated increasingly "intrapsychic" viewpoints. For example, constructivist ideas, currently of much interest to cognitive and systems theories, presuppose notions of internal representational narratives that serve to organize behavior and cognitive attributions in the external world. That one's underlying psychological state has paramount meaning in psychological (i.e., affective, behavioral, and cognitive) life is old news to psychoanalytic theory but relatively new news to many other modalities.

The concept of *transference* is central to a psychodynamic understanding of the way human beings function relationally. It embodies the assumption that we form early and enduring (though not immutable) representations of significant objects (i.e., usually people) that provide the templates by which we relate to later objects. This relation to later objects always reflects an admixture of the transferential templates and current relational data. Thus transference, and especially its broader cousin, mental representations, is quite analogous to the cognitive and developmental concept of *schema*. While addressing fundamentally similar ideas, transference incorporates issues of content over structure, and schema incorporates issues of structure over content. In other words, transference is a form of mental model that is dominated by the particular relationship content of the transference, be it authoritarian maternal, nurturant paternal, etc. Cognitive schemas are invoked primarily as denoting the way in which an important category of information is encoded, processed, and retrieved, with the specific content of that structure secondary. Nonetheless, the concept of transference, which is always relational, and schema, when used relationally, are for the most part parallel in meaning.

The cognitive-behavioral notion of *graduated exposure* is not equivalent to the concept of transference, but it captures in alternative terms one of the central dynamics of a patient's developing transference toward a therapist and how this is used therapeutically. Graduated exposure refers to the progression from exposure to minimal anxiety-generating situations to exposure to situations that generate intense anxiety. The latter situations are ones in which there is a perception of little opportunity for escape and in which the provocation can be either the situation itself that generates anxiety (*in vivo* exposure) or the memory or image of the situation that generates anxiety (imaginal exposure). The conceptual overlap here is that in analyzing the transference in psychoanalysis and insight-oriented psychotherapy, a therapist, through the treatment boundary and the application of technical neutrality, allows the patient to be gradually exposed to an intensifying transference reaction. This multifaceted reaction can then be used as a tool in analyzing the patient's character style, defensive structure, drive derivatives, etc. The transference exposure is both *in vivo* and imaginal, with the real aspects of the therapist and associated attributions interacting with the imaginal and fantasied aspects of earlier relational experience that are projected onto the therapist.

Therapeutic alliance is a concept that underlies all forms of productive psychotherapy, although its origin and usage is primarily within the psychodynamic perspective. A central reason for this is that psychodynamic psychotherapy, particularly psychoanalysis and insight-oriented therapy, makes explicit use of the therapeutic relation as a technical tool, and hence the vicissitudes of the therapeutic alliance are especially crucial. In behavioral and cognitive terminology, there are two concepts that capture aspects of the alliance; positive attribution and modeling.

Positive attribution addresses the idea that developing a positive transference is a fundamental element in a good working alliance. Whether one allows the positive transference to expand or makes it a subject of interpretation so as to diminish it, in all forms of dynamic psychotherapy there is utility in some degree of positive transference toward promoting an alliance between therapist and patient. Our contention is that the process of positive attribution toward the therapist is a conceptual parallel of positive transference. Another aspect of the therapeutic alliance is the likelihood that a patient will use the therapist as a model for adaptive ego and superego functioning. Hence, the notion of modeling as a form of *in vivo* learning is relevant. In this context modeling can be viewed as analogous to identification, which is another important component of a good therapeutic alliance. *Modeling* involves an extinction of a current behavior (or affect or cognition) through vicarious learning (i.e., observation) associated with the therapist. To put this less mechanistically, through the course of the initial sessions in a productive psychotherapy, as in the early moments of any relationship, the patient is especially receptive to learning from and about the therapist. If the quality of the relationship is appropriately supportive and boundaried, the patient will usually receive the range of verbal and nonverbal communications from the therapist with some openness, albeit perhaps at an unconscious level. These communications then become internalized to some extent and reidentified with as if they were one's own.

As almost any psychodynamic clinician can attest, *working through* constitutes the core of a psychotherapy and is one of the hardest of all ideas to conceptualize. We believe this is because working through, while seemingly referring to a circumscribed technique, actually reflects a multidetermined process in psycho-therapy wherein therapist and patient systematically apply and reapply the fundamentals of the clinical formulation and thera-peutic technique relevant for that particular patient, with the goal of effecting intrapsychic and/or functional improvement. It is inevitably difficult, then, to define working through given that it reflects the (re)application of a different amalgam of tech-niques and understandings for each patient. An easier defini-tional approach to working through might be to think of the de-sired end product of the working through process, which again is idiosyncratic to each patient but may encompass something within the domain of improved ego functioning, increased in-sight, symptomatic relief, better sublimatory outlets, and in-creased ability for both autonomy and relatedness. There are several cognitive and behavioral concepts that represent paral-lels to this domain.

Self-efficacy, a term consistent with cognitive psychology yet also having a generally recognizable meaning, refers to the abil-ity of an individual to be able to act in the world in a productive and self-motivated fashion. It is an omnibus construct that would be associated with any successful working through process. With-in a behavioral approach, *stimulus control* refers to the process by which one structures the psychological stressors in the environ-ment, and *contingency management* refers to the rewards and pun-ishments one invokes in order to regulate one's behavior. The ability to make use of both of these concepts is quite similar to the psychodynamic notion of good ego functioning and sublima-tory outlets, wherein one uses the full range of adaptive defenses in order to manage internal and external stressors. Finally, *cogni-tive self-monitoring* is a process in cognitive therapy where one develops skills at tracking the anticipatory, concurrent, and re-sulting cognitions associated with symptomatic distress. It is as-sociated with the fundamental psychodynamic therapeutic goal of increased insight.

Within the realm of *ego defense mechanisms,* there are several areas of overlap between cognitive theory and psychodynamic theory, particularly regarding the defenses of rationalization, projection, suppression, and repression. *Rationalization* refers to the process by which conflictual material is cognitively/

affectively reworked and consciously "justified" so as to recast the conflict in a less distressing way. It is a very frequently used mechanism and has a direct parallel to the notion of *cognitive reconstrual*, in which one takes on a constructivist stance toward conflictual "truths," reconstruing them in an alternative and more palatable way. *Projection* implies an ascribing of an unacceptable idea, affect, or impulse within oneself to another person, with the goal of "ridding" the self of any potential conflict associated with the idea/affect/impulse. Projection is analogous to the cognitive notion of *external attribution,* wherein one attributes the cause of something originating within oneself to someone or something outside oneself. The defense of *suppression,* which involves a conscious inattention to something intrapsychic that may be conflictual, is related to the more universal concept of *avoidance* of distressing stimuli. Finally, *repression,* a cornerstone notion in psychoanalytic theory, refers to the means by which an unacceptable or conflictual idea is driven from consciousness and available only unconsciously or in signal form consciously. This concept is similar to the idea of *exclusion of information,* whereby one defensively excludes potentially disturbing information that may lead to internal conflict. It is not truly analogous to repression, in that repression implies an unconscious process, something which is not addressed in cognitive or behavioral theories. Exclusion of information is a process by which cognitively dissonant information is "nipped in the bud" prior to being encoded and processed.

A final area of conceptual overlap to be discussed concerns the processes of psychodynamic interpretation (i.e., explanation of meanings), which include *clarification, confrontation,* and *interpretation proper.* Clarification refers to the beginning and most frequent part of the interpretive process, when a therapist focuses on elucidating the various aspects of a patient's experience of the current material being discussed in session. It is aimed at expanding the patient's and therapist's respective awarenesses of the patient's material. The next level of interpretation is confrontation, in which a therapist points out areas of inconsistency between aspects of the patient's presented content, or between content and affects or motivations—in other words, engaging the patient in critical questioning of discrepancies in manifest or intrapsychic content. This level of interpretation serves to increase observing ego and begins to bring more conflictual material into consciousness. The last level of the process is interpretation proper, wherein a therapist offers explanations or attributions of meaning to some aspect of the patient's material. Interpretations usually involve some explanation of the origin or presumed motivating factors of intrapsychic conflict.

These three levels of the interpretive process have an interesting parallel with three techniques for effecting change in negative cognitions as outlined by Craighead, Craighead, Kazdin, and Mahoney (1994): "(1) *distancing* (teaching the client to re-evaluate ingrained beliefs and judgments by making them more explicit and testing their validity); (2) *decentering* (getting clients to see that they are not the focus of all events); (3) *reattribution* (getting clients to change their attributional style)" (p. 43). Without being too redundant, it is worth pointing out that both the psychodynamic model of interpretation and the cognitive model of correcting negative cognitions share the fundamental element of perspective building. Clarification and distancing approach perspective building by bringing increased material into awareness and thereby making it more available for examination. Confrontation and decentering both ask patients to take a step backward and view their material from more than one angle. Interpretation proper and reattribution both engage patients in re-evaluating the meanings they ascribe to their external and intrapsychic "realities."

WHY SHOULD I SPEAK THEIR LANGUAGE?

Having read through the material of this chapter, you might well be reacting with increasing resentment. When we have discussed this material with colleagues, many take it in with understanding and a sense of relief that areas of theoretical convergence and functionality are being described so concretely; others react with anger and such questions as "Why should I have to speak 'their' language rather than they understanding mine?" The answer is twofold. The first is a pragmatic one. Managed care is a financially driven management technique aimed at reducing costs.

Given this perspective, it is not surprising that it should have developed more comfort with those modalities of treatment (i.e., behavioral and cognitive) whose language is closer to that of symptoms and functionality and which are generally shorter-term than psychodynamic psychotherapy. So the first reason to speak more of "their" language, which is an amalgam of behavioral, cognitive, and functional terminology, is that this has become the dominant language of managed care. The second reason to develop more familiarity with their language is that it will promote the kind of comfort with psychodynamics that will then allow them to learn more of the efficacy of psychodynamic treatments, for which we should also advocate. Comfort makes for easier communication and the motivation to learn another perspective. Being true to psychodynamic treatment principles does not preclude communicating these principles in language that is more understandable to a nonpsychodynamic audience, as long as you are not misrepresenting your work as other than it really is. What this means in practice is that to reflexively substitute all of the behavioral/cognitive/functional concepts for psychodynamic concepts in verbal or written communication would be a misrepresentation; to use a few of the concepts judiciously and appropriately in the context of describing a psychodynamic treatment will dramatically enhance the accessibility of your communication and make authorization much more likely.

5

Documenting Psychodynamic Treatment in a Managed Care Format

Virtually every psychodynamic psychotherapist who makes use of third-party insurance reimbursement has by now become inundated with requests for documentation of his/her work in order to gain further authorization for therapy sessions. While time consuming, of questionable utility, and often seemingly trivial, another source of resistance for psychodynamic clinicians arises from the fact that there can be a huge gap between the questions being asked (and consequently what is used as a basis for evaluation of the treatment) and the actual work going on in the therapy. This process then leads many psychodynamic clinicians to the erroneous belief that under the best of conditions they will still be unlikely to secure authorization for psychodynamic work. Building upon the conceptual foundation presented in Chapter Four, this chapter addresses the issue of how to write outpatient treatment plans and updates that are consistent with psychodynamic work yet simultaneously formulated in functional language, and hence both acceptable to managed care companies and effective in gaining authorization.[1]

When a therapist writes up a case psychodynamically, there are several elements usually covered. In addition to the requisite demographic, presenting problem, history, and mental status data, there is an attempt to understand and explain a patient's symptoms in the context of his/her early relational history, predominant intrapsychic conflicts, defensive constellation, sublimatory channels, and quality of current object relations. In writing up a case for a managed care company, however, there is little need to explicitly focus on these latter areas of psychodynamic interest, even though there remains a need for the therapist to understand and intervene with the patient based on these areas of interest. *The therapist's task is to inform the managed care organization of enough history and current symptoms to make the discussion of functional impairment clear and plausible.* As we noted earlier, functional impairment is the overarching benchmark in managed care, with intrapsychic impairment important but secondary. So, for example, if a 24-year-old male patient appears to you to be unconsciously struggling with a maternal representation that leads him to expect scolding and "unfair" demands from his girlfriends, and characteristically reacts to this with passive–aggressive withdrawal and conflict avoidance, this patient's psychodynamics might argue for a moderate-term dynamic psychotherapy organized around the conflictual maternal representation. To seek authorization from a managed care company for this treatment, a written focus on this intrapsychic conflict would likely be ineffective, but by focusing on the *functional analogues* of the same conflict (i.e., repeated inability to sustain an intimate relationship; significant relational distress that impairs concentration at work), treatment authorization would be likely.

To review, when writing up a psychodynamic case from a functional perspective, the first step is still to develop, but not document, a psychodynamic formulation. The next step is to document the problem-

---

[1]The case material presented in this chapter has been contributed, in part, by Andrea Allen, PhD, and Pauline Bergstein, PhD. Names, histories, and clinical descriptions have been disguised to protect confidentiality.

atic/symptomatic functional manifestations of the dynamic conflict(s). This latter step is the one of interest to a managed care organization. When writing up a case organized around functional abilities, there are several essential elements to be included, as outlined in Table 2. These elements are not universal, in that each managed care organization has its own version of an outpatient treatment report. There does tend to be much overlap in the basic categories, and the table presents a prototypical outline.

The first element consists of a few bits of basic demographic information, with name and social security (or member identification) number being the most important of these. Almost all managed care organizations use the social security number as the record-keeping access vehicle, and it is a necessity for all patients. The presenting problem section should include a statement of problems as close to the patient's wording as possible; patient's needs and the degree to which these are met are important markers of treatment success from the managed care organization's perspective. Current mental status and diagnosis should be brief but complete—a full five-axis DSM-IV diagnosis (which includes a Global Assessment of Functioning score) is usually required. The next section, current functional level, is where one

---

TABLE 2. Prototypical Outpatient Treatment Report Format

Identifying information: Patient's name, address, phone, employer, Social Security number, and date of birth; insured's employer and Social Security number (if different from patient's)

Presenting problems (as stated by the patient)

Brief relevant history (include any history of prior treatment for this patient, as well as any family psychiatric history)

Current mental status and diagnosis (DSM-IV)

Current functional level (including work, education, family and friendships, and independent living)

Treatment goals, therapeutic modalities, and time estimated to reach each goal

Number of sessions requested (for both current authorization and the overall anticipated treatment)

Therapist information: Therapist's name, signature, Social Security number, license number

---

documents the clear functional limitations that will justify treatment. These must also be consistent with the diagnosis given. The treatment goals established should be focused and associated with the functional deficits. For each treatment goal, there should also be notation of the therapeutic modality or specific interventions to be used, and often there is a request for a time estimate to reach the goal(s). This material then often leads to a request for both a current and overall number of treatment sessions to be authorized. It is important that the overall number of sessions anticipated by the therapist be realistic and appropriate to the nature of the problems being addressed in the treatment plan. (Not all managed care organizations ask the therapist to request a specific number of sessions; some automatically authorize a predefined number of sessions following each review as long as the treatment plan continues to be certified.) It is tempting for some therapists to make consistently large requests, assuming that these will be cut down to some extent but still greater than if one were to request a smaller number. This is ultimately a bad tactic, as the managed care organization may view a therapist's requests as untrustworthy and stop referring patients, and/or not evaluate treatment requests critically. This can become especially problematic when a therapist does indeed need to secure a greater number of sessions for certain patients whose clinical presentation demands it. Finally, all treatment requests must include the therapist's name, signature (with degree), social security number and/or provider number for that organization, and often license number as well.

More than anything, the treatment plan should be accurate, brief, and to the point, in language that the reviewer will understand. Remember that the task of the report is to give a reviewer just enough information to be able to ascertain whether treatment is indicated as proposed, not to develop a full enough understanding of the patient to be able to really understand the patient's problems. This is tough for many clinicians, since we are generally used to discussing our work in appropriate depth with others who are either collateral providers or interested colleagues. Notwithstanding the need for brevity, the treatment plan should be compatible with psychodynamic treatment in a largely functional language.

To make this discussion clearer, we will first present an example of a brief case history and formulation on intake, written from a psychodynamic perspective, followed by a formulation of this same case within a format more useful to a managed care context. The form and content of this first version of the case, as with most psychodynamic formulations, aims to maximally inform the reader about relevant dynamics and treatment questions, not to gain treatment authorization from a third party. The second version of the case should read as compatible with the first but appear more frugal in the amount of information given, and much more functional than dynamic in its language.

INTAKE REPORTS

Psychodynamic Formulation

PRESENTING PROBLEM

Molly is a 37-year-old woman who has presented for psychotherapy. At the first of two intake sessions she complained of a depressed mood accompanied by irritability and exhaustion due to chronic marital conflict and financial distress. She states that her marital problems with her husband have been exacerbated by his chronic unemployment and the resultant financial pressure placed upon her. When originally asked about her expectations for the future of the marriage, she expressed much ambivalence and indecision and stated that "I'm starting to feel like I've been wasting my life [with him]."

HISTORY

This is a first marriage for Molly and the second for her spouse. The couple is childless by choice. Molly stated that she felt that there were both communication and trust problems from early on in her 8-year marriage. She has described her progressive disillusionment with her husband and her growing feeling that "life was passing her by" due to the encumbrances of her relationship.

Molly claims that she never expected to be married and admitted to being a "man hater." She hypothesized that this resulted from her experience of her father, who was described as untrustworthy, "a womanizer," "a pathological liar," and who was for the most part "absent" from the family. Her mother was described as a "yeller and a hitter" but the "strength" of the family. Molly is the third of five siblings, stating that "I grew up unloved and on my own" and that she "lived in secrets" because her "chaotic" family lived in such a small house that the children were forced to keep their thoughts, problems, and emotions to themselves.

PERSONALITY DYNAMICS

The tone of Molly's conversation is most often calm and soft spoken, her words are carefully chosen, and her conversation flows in an unhurried, almost methodical pace. She expresses herself well and exhibits a high degree of intellectual curiosity. Her responses to questions are very detail laden and systematically presented. It is important to note that the content of the patient's conversation is almost exclusively about others and not herself. Therapist efforts to redirect conversation to the patient are often met with passive resistance. Also, Molly exhibits a limited range of affect, showing little emotional reactivity to changes in conversational theme. At times when she does begin to express emotion, she quickly changes the path of the conversation. It is only in the most recent sessions that Molly has, after much prodding, admitted to feelings of anger or rage, or allowed her eyes to well with tears for a moment or two.

Molly impresses as an individual who strives to create order from disorder and who approaches most elements in her life in a highly intellectualized, systematic manner. Her style is to "talk (and think) things out," in an apparent effort to avoid feelings, and is suggestive of an obsessive personality style. In a classical psychoanalytic perspective, Molly's obsessive-compulsive style can be framed in terms of an anal character type, with the relevant dynamics representative of anal-sadism. In support of this conceptualization, there is strong indication of deep, repressed internalized hostility in this individual. There also appear to be identity and dependency issues that are characteristic of this character type.

Consistent with psychodynamic theory, this obsessive individual presents with a counterdependent posture in compensation for severe feelings of self-doubt and ambivalence concerning relational issues and authority figures, and a corresponding negativistic outlook. It is interesting that when asked what she would like from her husband, her answer was "to be acknowledged." Molly seems greatly disenfranchised in her ability to acknowledge or see value in herself.

The picture of the moral self-control that typifies the self-punishing depressive superego appears to be, in part, reflective of Molly's character structure. She presents as having chronic depression, as represented by exhaustion, work, and marital difficulties, that she attributes ultimately to her own shortcomings in relational contexts. Specifically, she cites as reasons for her depression both her long-term inability to address her feelings concerning the condition of her marriage, and her indecisiveness concerning its future. In addition, she expresses ambivalence with authority figures (including almost everyone at the company that employs her), appears overly conscientious in her work yet simultaneously tardy many mornings, and is easily disappointed with herself and others.

It is also noteworthy that, although she has admitted to feeling comfortable with the therapist, Molly has maintained what can be described as a conflicted, varying emotional distance and has only allowed a preliminary positive connection to grow very slowly. This behavior seems representative of the conflicts concerning trust, independence, and personal distance characteristic of the anal stage of development.

DEFENSIVE STYLE

According to psychodynamic theory, an anaclitic depressive style, as currently exhibited by Molly, is in part rooted in an undercurrent of hate that creates ambivalence in loving relationships. Such ambivalence has roots in early childhood, where love and care were made contingent upon compliance and expressions of hate were suppressed. The felt hostility is then turned against the self and causes exaggerated guilt. The "danger" now comes from within; hence, the depressive may adopt a stance of appeasing others as a palliative for the activation of self-hatred. This dynamic is particularly descriptive of Molly's developmental and interpersonal history, the support for which is not so much in Molly's sense of guilt but in her sense of responsibility for her marriage (e.g., she regards the problems as her "fault" because she could not "teach [her husband] enough to make it work"). This posture is especially poignant in the context of the litany of reported abuses and acts of selfishness by the husband that Molly recounted to the therapist. Also, as mentioned, Molly is self-disparaging concerning her talents and achievements—the message continually delivered is one of being "never good enough."

As repression and denial fail her, as it appears each of these defenses has done with increasing frequency through the course of her marriage, introjection tends to become the predominant defense. If we assume that introjection is developmentally based on oral incorporation, it is interesting to note that approximately 3 years ago, when Molly first realized that her marriage was failing, she quickly began to put on excess weight and continues to do so. We may hypothesize that this oral incorporation coincides with the failure of repression to counter her relational troubles and therefore the decline of perceived narcissistic supplies. She ate to fill this void, as well as to service the internalized self-hatred.

When under psychic stress due to the fact that her other defenses have broken down, her defensive posture regresses through the use of somatization. She states that at times of stress her arthritis will flare up, her blood pressure will become conspicuously high, or she will "just get sick." Her tendency to use somatization is another example of her likelihood of turning anger upon herself rather than others.

The most primitive of Molly's defenses is her primary egocentrism or omnipotent control, which accompanies her belief that the success or failure of the marriage is her fault. At the core of many of her thought processes is the belief that, either at work or home, she could have changed things had she "thought it out" better. This leads to Molly's most frequently used and observable defense, intellectualization, which she frequently employs in conjunction with isolation. As already described, Molly thinks her way through her life in order not to feel and in order not to be caught "off guard." It appears that the more her life turns out differently than she had planned, the more she compensates by trying to think, plan, and anticipate.

TREATMENT FOCUS

Given the depth and breadth of the intrapsychic conflicts presented by Molly, an insight-oriented psychotherapy is indicated. However, given the limitations of her financial and insurance situations, a once-per-week psychotherapy has been initiated with both an expressive and, where appropriate, ego-supportive focus. Although Molly presents her marriage as the identified problem, the therapist will also slowly attempt to have Molly focus on herself, her conflicts, and her needs. The goal is to increase her identity as a self-advocate rather than as a caretaker and to enable her to be fundamentally self-supporting, or at least not self-defeating. In addition, it is clear that even with a wide repertoire of available defenses, her adaptive defenses are failing. A goal of treatment will be to reinforce Molly's adaptive defenses and help her to gain knowledge of the defended-against dynamic conflicts, thereby mitigating the impact these long-standing conflicts exert in her current life.

This psychodynamic formulation offers a rich description of the patient's life situation, central dynamics and areas of conflict, and treatment prospects. It is written to both inform and interest the reader, engaging in a thoughtful examination of the complications of an individual's developmental history in the context of external reality. The material as written, however, would be unlikely to gain treatment authorization from a managed care organization. For this purpose, it is too verbose, conceptual, and—most significantly—rooted in language that a reviewer would have difficulty understanding. Without altering the fundamental formulation or treatment goals, this same clinical data can be reframed in a language and form that a managed care reviewer would find accessible. To rework this material within a functional context, the form outlined in Table 2 will be used. It offers a prototypical outpatient treatment report structure that queries the specific type of information that managed care organizations are interested in receiving:

Outpatient Treatment Report

IDENTIFYING INFORMATION

Name of Patient: Molly K.
Address: 251 N. Arlington Street, Oakville, MO, 64237
Phone: (802) 872-3697   **Employer:** Birchwood Industries
Soc. Sec. #: 258-84-7389   **Date of Birth:** 7/3/56

PRESENTING PROBLEMS

Ms. K. began treatment 6 weeks ago, complaining of a depressed mood accompanied by irritability and exhaustion due to chronic marital conflict and financial distress. She attributes the marital stressors to her husband's chronic unemployment and the resultant financial pressures on her, and states that "I'm starting to feel like I've been wasting my life [with him]."

BRIEF RELEVANT HISTORY

This is a first marriage for Ms. K., and the second for her spouse. The couple is childless by choice. The patient stated that she felt that there were both communication and trust problems from early on in her 8-

year marriage, with a growing uncertainty about continuing the relationship. She also reports chronic distrust of men, which she attributes to a chaotic early family life.

CURRENT MENTAL STATUS AND DIAGNOSIS (DSM-IV)

Mental status revealed a dysthymic mood, with slightly constricted affect. Speech was slow and methodical, with obsessional content. Suicidal/homicidal ideation was denied. All other indicators were within normal limits.

Axis I   – 300.4 Dysthymic Disorder
        – V61.1 Partner Relational Problem
Axis II – 301.4 Obsessive-Compulsive Personality Disorder
Axis III – history of benign ovarian cysts
Axis IV – marital and financial distress
Axis V   – (1) Current GAF: 62
        – (2) Highest GAF, past year: 70

CURRENT FUNCTIONAL LEVEL

The central functional deficits for Ms. K. center around depression and obsessionalism. The depression is manifest in limited affective responsiveness, subjective complaints of depressed mood, mild psychomotor retardation, reduced work efficiency, and difficulty mobilizing herself in the mornings. Her attribution of depression to the many current stressors, especially the distressed marital relationship, appears to be accurate. Additionally, the patient appears to use obsessional thinking in order to cognitively reconstrue and avoid affectively disturbing experiences/memories. The obsessionalism manifests in quite verbose, overly systematic descriptions of her experiences, a reported and observable tendency to vigilantly think through and try to anticipate any possibly distressing future outcomes, and the mistaken attribution that if she thought things through better at work and home she could block any negative outcomes.

TREATMENT GOALS, THERAPEUTIC MODALITIES, AND TIME ESTIMATED TO REACH EACH GOAL

1. Evaluate severity of depression, and need for psychopharmacological intervention—3 weeks.

2. Allow for fuller expression of excluded negative affects regarding marital situation—3 months.

3. Identify alternative action plans regarding marital distress; consider couple therapy referral—2 months.

4. Challenge and guide the patient in reconstruing her negative self-attributions, promoting improved self-monitoring skills—5 months.

5. Improve the patient's awareness of dysfunctional relational patterns and ability to employ alternative patterns—5 months.

6. Consider referral to women's support group or depression self-help group—1 month.

The treatment modality employed to reach the above goals will blend interpersonal/supportive and cognitive techniques. The patient has participated in and is cooperative with this treatment plan, and prognosis is considered good.

NUMBER OF SESSIONS REQUESTED

Current treatment request—12 sessions; Estimated overall treatment length to reach goals—30 sessions

Therapist Information
Therapist's Name: Signature:
Soc. Sec. #:   **License Number:**

There are several points of contrast between the psychodynamic and functional write-ups of this clinical material, the most obvious of which is the length. The psychodynamic write-up is twice the length of the functional one; brevity has traditionally been viewed as inappropriately reductive for psychodynamic work, as is reflected in the thoughtful documentation of such work. Yet one can, and should, in a managed care format, reasonably document clinical work in less space and detail, especially given the goal of treatment authorization versus treatment information. This involves a cognitive reconstrual in the mindset of the therapist from collegial consultation to "just-sufficient information," the latter of which is the task at hand when requesting authorization. To present just sufficient information, which reduces complicated clinical information to minimal yet meaningful parts, doesn't invalidate the richness of the actual treatment situation. *Your task is to incorporate this richness into your interventions with the patient in your office; the reviewer need only feel confident that you are aware of the parameters involved and can communicate and intervene within these parameters effectively and efficiently.*

These two versions of the write-up additionally introduce several key points governing treatment documentation for managed care organizations:

1. *The primacy of functioning.* Treatment reviewers focus on functional ability above all else. Insight is only relevant in the documentation to the extent that it directly improves functional ability. Therefore, while insight is a central therapeutic tool in many psychodynamic treatments, stick with documenting the functional analogues in most cases, not the potential value of insight per se.

2. *Treatment focus.* Document expected changes in symptoms and behavior rather than focusing on internal structural change or object relational improvements. Again, structural and object relational change usually produces symptomatic relief, and this is the eventual target goal of most treatments. Of course, with some patients (e.g., those using repressive defenses) challenging the defensive structure can temporarily produce a worsening in symptoms before a diminution. If this is the case, present a clear rationale that demonstrates the necessity of a systematic treatment plan with symptomatic relief as the eventual (and not too far-off) goal.

3. *Don't use highly technical language.* Given the diversity in the training of reviewers, use clear and either cognitive-behavioral or theoretically neutral functional language to describe psychodynamic interventions. Such language is most likely to be interpretable by all, not just those well trained in psychodynamics.

4. *Goals/progress/outcome/prognosis.* Every treatment presented for review should be firmly anchored in these four areas. Other historical or formulative material should be added where appropriate, but stick with the basics first. Demonstrate a goal-oriented approach that is consistent with the diagnosis, document progress made toward those goals, make clear what your benchmarks are for evaluating outcome, and always offer a prognostic assessment.

FOLLOW-UP TREATMENT REPORTS

This last issue of evaluating outcome is relevant for initial write-ups of cases as well as for treatment updates. While treatment updates contain much of the same information as the initial outpatient treatment report, there is generally less emphasis on history and more on treatment progress and goal attainment and/or new goals. It is important to demonstrate (and believe) that you take the goals seriously and realistically evaluate progress toward attainment, preferably with behavioral markers. This may sound like yet another behavioral sellout to managed care. In fact, enacting behavioral change as a result of intrapsychic change has traditionally been the litmus test for termination in brief dynamic therapy. To a managed care organization, as well as to clinical researchers in personality assessment, evaluating and trusting measures of intrapsychic change is problematic at best. Projective measures provide the richest data, and perhaps the most useful to a dynamic clinician, but such data are not generally reliable across patients or across scorers. Behavioral sequelae to intrapsychic change are much more easily conveyed to and trusted by managed care reviewers. Even better from their perspective, and useful clinically, are reports that document ongoing evaluation of treatment progress using standardized psychological measures. In Chapter Seven we take up in detail the variety of available measures and how one makes appropriate choices among them. For now, we will illustrate another contrast between a psychodynamic and a functional formulation, but this time for a treatment that has already been underway for several months. As earlier, we first present the psychodynamic formulation, which offers a relatively full history and description of the patient's treatment progress, followed by a treatment update more suitable to a managed care context.

Psychodynamic Formulation

PRESENTING PROBLEM

Selena is a 57-year-old woman from Chile who has been living in the city for approximately 2 years. A physician at a local hospital who was treating her for medical problems referred her to the Center for Community Services (CCS) in September due to depression. The patient came to CCS complaining of being depressed, crying all the time, having trouble sleeping, fatigue, nervousness, having trouble concentrating and making decisions, and feeling very discouraged about her life. She reported wanting to be by herself and not wanting to have to see anyone because recent conflicts she'd been having with a son and daughter-in-law wiped her out for days. In addition, she reported having flashbacks of childhood sexual abuse as well as intrusive thoughts regarding the murder of a son and other difficult losses. She reported multiple medical difficulties including headaches, gastrointestinal difficulties (cause unknown), and back pain.

HISTORY

Selena has had a history of depression, including an inpatient hospitalization in 1976. Several losses and interpersonal conflicts seem to have precipitated her current crisis.

In 1993, while Selena was still living in Chile, a 12-year-old grandson whom she had raised since infancy (a son of one of her sons) was kidnapped by his mother and taken to live in another country. At the time Selena began treatment, she was unable to reach them by phone and had been getting no response to her letters. She was distraught over this loss and worried about what was happening to the boy: "I don't know if he's being properly looked after, if he's enrolled in school."

In late 1993, the patient came to the city to live with one of her adult sons in order to help him by taking care of his two young children while he and his wife worked. Conflict quickly developed between the patient and her daughter-in-law which, after about a year, resulted in the patient moving out. She went to stay temporarily with a friend from South America and the woman's three children. In this apartment, Selena had to share a room with a rebellious teenage girl, which resulted in her having no privacy, no peace and quiet, and the theft of her jewelry and other belongings. She was supposed to be paid to take care of the children; however, the patient reported that the woman never lived up to their agreement, resulting in constant conflict.

In addition, Selena felt humiliated by her lack of success in this move to the city. She had hoped to be able to help her son, have the rewards of caring for her grandchildren, and make some money on the side which she hoped to use to help some of her other grandchildren. She can't face "going back home to Chile empty-handed because we're proud people." So, she was stuck in the city living in a very stressful situation, with increasing health problems, in poverty, living on minimal welfare and Medicaid, and with few family members and friends to help her.

Her background predisposes her to depression and interpersonal and intrapsychic conflict. The patient was reportedly a victim of chronic sexual abuse (from age 3 to 13) at the hands of an adult male relative. She told no one because she believed he had the confidence of her parents and had convinced them that she was very disobedient and dishonest—was often put in charge of disciplining her—and said that if she told anyone they'd never believe her and he'd punish her. She was also sexually abused on isolated occasions by other adult male relatives. In addition, at age 13, after being raped by the male relative near a country road and left alone, a stranger who had observed the rape came up and raped her himself. None of these events was revealed to anyone until recently.

The patient has five children, four of whom are still living: two sons (one in the city, one back in Chile) and two daughters (in the Midwest). She has at least five grandchildren. She has had no contact with the father of her children for over 20 years.

Over the past 15 years the patient suffered several difficult losses. Her father died; her middle child, an 18-year-old son, was murdered; this was followed by her mother's death. Also, a friend was shot to death in a club—for which she feels guilty since he wouldn't have been there if she hadn't sent him away, saying she was too tired to talk to him that night. In addition, a brother of hers was murdered, and his son was also murdered 2 years later.

PERSONALITY DYNAMICS AND DEFENSIVE STYLE

Selena's central defenses are reaction formation and turning against the self. She has focused her life on taking care of others (i.e., reaction formation). She has spent most of her adult life raising her children, their children, and the children of various friends and neighbors who were unable or unavailable to raise them. This may be seen as a defense against unconscious anger and dependency needs aroused by her abusive childhood—an attempt to correctively "reparent" herself through multiple other parenting relationships. Although the patient is openly very angry toward the man (now deceased) who abused her, she is completely unaware of any feelings of anger toward her parents, who did not protect her during this time. She speaks of them very fondly and, most notably, took on responsibility for nursing each of them through long illnesses prior to their deaths.

Reaction formation has in some ways been an adaptive defense. Despite her stated desire to be alone, she has received much satisfaction from taking care of children and remains close to many of them today. It has become clear that she does have many meaningful interpersonal ties and most are more rewarding and more reciprocal than the ones that have been predominant in the last year or two. Nonetheless, her style of relating leaves her vulnerable to not having her own needs met, since she does not let her needs be known and simply hopes that people will guess what they are and fulfill them. In addition, she is unable to protect herself from loss. For example, she seems to have opened her home and heart repeatedly to children for years at a time only to have them taken away from her when their parents want them back. This is not something she has been able to easily bounce back from.

She also turns some of this unresolved conflict against herself, which promotes cycles of strong depressive symptoms. She is almost never able to express anger toward others or to foresee her own vulnerability and protect herself. Instead she repeatedly places herself in situations where she can be victimized. These problems reflect defensive failures, because this vulnerability neither extends throughout all areas of her life nor reflects a basic lack of cognitive or other skills. For example, she can be an extremely effective businesswoman, especially if it is to benefit someone else, yet she hasn't been able to get the results of medical tests she underwent 8 months ago.

As the stress she is under increases, the patient tends to somatize, expressing her intrapsychic conflict and external stresses through multiple physical complaints. The patient has spent years suppressing her thoughts and feelings regarding her abuse and has not fully confronted the major losses in her life, including the murder of her son.

TREATMENT PROGRESS

Selena began therapy 8 months ago and has attended 18 sessions of psychotherapy to date. Her attendance has recently been very regular, but it has been limited somewhat by her health problems and was interrupted twice for several weeks when she visited her son in Chile and then her daughters in the Midwest. She was referred for antidepressant medication early on in her treatment but saw a psychiatrist who "upset" her and she wouldn't go back. She recently saw a different psychiatrist and just began taking Zoloft (sertraline).

Therapy has been supportive in nature. The focus has been on encouraging the patient's efforts to take care of and consider her own needs and improve her family relationships. This has been done in ways which strengthen the positive aspects of the patient's self-image and defensive structure. For example, taking more account of her own needs is framed in the context of this being good for her children or grandchildren (to encourage their own development or provide a role model, etc.).

The patient arrived in therapy believing that her problems stemmed, in large part, from her childhood sexual abuse and her tendency to try to suppress the thoughts and feelings these experiences arouse. In therapy, links have been pointed out between these experiences and her tendency to accept poor treatment from others and allow herself to be victimized. This has been used to help her begin to learn new ways of protecting herself without her feeling selfish or cold. Therapy has helped her to improve her efforts to clarify her expectations of those she's interacting with and to be direct about her needs and expectations. The focus on understanding and improving her current relationships, such as making her communications more clear, direct and less passive, have resulted in changes in her thoughts and feelings about her relationships, but there has been no noticeable change in her problematic enduring relationships. She is, however, spending less time with those individuals and more with those who are more supportive and appreciative of her. As a result of all of these gains, her need for reaction formation and turning against the self has diminished, and so her depression as a consequence of unresolved conflict and repressed anger has become less intense.

The patient's living situation has also improved. She has moved in with a female relative, as well as the female relative's husband and mother-in-law, and their several children. The female relative's hope was that Selena would provide company for the mother-in-law, who seems to be a very difficult woman. While Selena occasionally takes care of the children, she has no formal responsibilities within the household and has her own room. Her only conflicts within this household are with the mother-in-law, but these are tolerable because the woman drives everyone crazy so the patient feels supported.

She has made the decision that she wants to return to Chile and no longer seems so haunted by thoughts of going home empty-handed or humiliated, except that she does not want to return until she can pay her own airfare. Actually, her son in Chile would rather just pay it himself and have her back safely, but she wants very much not to feel dependent.

Although the patient began therapy talking about her sexual abuse and the need to deal with it, in sessions she has tended to focus on current problems. At this time, because her emotional state has improved, the question of whether or not she wants to more fully deal with/explore her experiences of sexual abuse will be discussed further with the patient. Such work would likely require a considerable time and emotional commitment on Selena's part.

The material of this psychodynamic write-up of an ongoing treatment case demonstrates a good working understanding of the relevant dynamic conflicts. Foremost among these are the conflicts resulting from early sexual abuse and a history of multiple significant losses, with a pattern of reaction formation and turning against the self as countervening defensive maneuvers. While supportive psychodynamic psychotherapy appears to have been useful to date in diminishing depressive symptoms and a self-defeating style, framing the gains and need for further treatment in dynamic terms would likely be met with "resistance" from a managed care reviewer. The write-up that follows reworks this case in a brief, functional language that is consistent with the psychodynamic formulation above, but puts the therapeutic work in alternative language. When reading it, remember that this report is an update on ongoing treatment, and presupposes that there has already been an original fuller write-up covering presenting problems and history:

Outpatient Treatment Update

IDENTIFYING INFORMATION

Name of Patient: Selena
Address: 22-76 Wallace Boulevard, Northfield, CA 58440
Phone: (419)395-3957   **Employer:** None (Medicaid)
Soc. Sec. #: 687-65-1294   **Date of Birth:** 11/28/36

PRESENTING PROBLEMS

The patient came to CCS complaining of being depressed, crying all the time, having trouble sleeping, fatigue, nervousness, having trouble concentrating and making decisions, and feeling very discouraged about her life. In addition, she reported flashbacks of childhood sexual abuse as well as intrusive thoughts regarding the murder of a son and several other difficult losses.

BRIEF RELEVANT HISTORY

No new history since last report.

CURRENT MENTAL STATUS AND DIAGNOSIS (DSM-IV)

Mental status reveals dysthymic episodes with no current major depressive symptomatology. Concentration has improved but still shows some impairment. Other indicators are within normal limits.

> **Axis I** — Major depressive disorder, recurrent, moderate (296.32)
> — Posttraumatic stress disorder (309.81)
> **Axis II** — None
> **Axis III** — Headaches, gastrointestinal difficulties, high cholesterol, allergies requiring restricted diet (note that patient has history of hypothyroidism)
> **Axis IV** — Housing problems, problem with primary social support group, financial problems, poor access to health care services
> **Axis V** — (1) Current GAF: 55
> — (2) Highest GAF, past year: 55

CURRENT FUNCTIONAL LEVEL

Patient unable to work due to history of periodic depression, flashbacks, intrusive thoughts, and health problems. Has conflictual relationships with family members which contribute to and are exacerbated by depression.

TREATMENT GOALS, THERAPEUTIC MODALITIES, AND TIME ESTIMATED TO REACH EACH GOAL

1. The patient has finally started taking antidepressant medication. Her clinical response will be monitored for possible side effects and compliance difficulties—12 weeks.
2. The patient will improve her assertiveness in getting results

of recent medical tests, and this behavior will generalize to other personal needs situations—6 weeks.

3. The patient has been expanding her network of positive (as opposed to self-defeating or abusive) social supports and will now seek supportive contact with a friend or relative outside her home at least three times per week—4 weeks.

4. Following on the patient's increased understanding of sources of problems in relationships with her children, she will develop and implement action plans to improve the quality of her interactions with at least two children or grandchildren—12 weeks.

5. The question of whether patient wants to work on her history of abuse, and its likely impact on current intrusive thoughts and somatic symptoms, will now be evaluated, as a sufficient therapeutic relationship has been established. Should she decide to do so, individual or group therapy resources to allow adequate time for this will be explored—6 weeks.

NUMBER OF SESSIONS REQUESTED

Current treatment request—12 sessions; sessions completed to date—18 sessions; estimated overall treatment length to reach goals—36 sessions

Therapist Information
Therapist's Name: Signature:
Soc. Sec. #:   **License Number:**

This second version of a treatment update has underscored the usefulness of documenting the status of prior interventions, as well as keeping repeated information, such as basic history, to a minimum. As with just about any service a consumer is receiving, both patients and managed care organization reviewers want to be assured that the service you are offering is needed and effective. The treatment update provides the opportunity to document this. It is not necessary to present a rosy picture of treatment, as if in some ideal universe all interventions were maximally effective and all patients improved in a steadily accelerating pattern. Managed care reviewers know that people and treatments are not perfect—they just need enough data and rationale to be assured that the treatment plan and progress toward it are reasonable and worthy of continued support.

6

Short-Term
Treatment Applications

Managed care generally limits the types of interventions we are able to implement. This manifests most conspicuously in an often strict regulation of the duration of treatment through dictating the number of approved sessions. While a small but growing body of research supports the cost and treatment effectiveness of long-term psychodynamic treatment in certain cases (e.g., Blatt, Ford, Berman, Cook, & Meyer, 1988; Lazar, 1997; Seligman & Levant, 1998), it can be helpful to explore a range of short-term dynamic psychotherapy variables. In doing so, we are not advocating mere acquiescence to the real or perceived temporal demands of managed care, but rather the capacity for adaptability. Again, it is our belief that by increasing awareness of potential treatment options, you will be able to approach managed care and the treatment situation from a more informed and empowered position. This will not only enable you to make responsible treatment decisions when faced with managed care constraints but also provide you with legitimate rationale to argue for additional sessions when appropriate. Furthermore, whether or not you are constrained by limitations imposed by managed care, short-term dynamic therapy has much to offer and, for some patients, may in fact be the treatment of choice.

Despite many recent innovations and a wide array of treatments considered "brief," there still remains a misconception among many clinicians that there is only one type of short-term dynamic psychotherapy, which dictates rather strict inclusion criteria. For instance, it is often assumed that patients must be high functioning and experiencing less severe psychopathology (e.g., an adjustment reaction to recent loss) to benefit from short-term treatment. *In actuality, there exist a variety of dynamically oriented short-term psychotherapies, from those with systematically defined structures and an ego-confrontive (insight-oriented) stance to those with less defined temporal structures and an ego-supportive stance.* In this chapter, we will present an overview of treatment grouping variables and then examine an illustrative case vignette highlighting the use of extratherapeutic transferences in a short-term psychodynamic treatment.

SHORT-TERM DYNAMIC THERAPY TREATMENT VARIABLES

Among the different types of short-term dynamic psychotherapies, there are several critical grouping variables which in some cases clearly differentiate that form of therapy from the others and in other cases apply simultaneously to several forms of therapy. These variables include the following:

1. The definition or lack of definition of the overall time boundaries of the treatment (i.e., maximum number of sessions)
2. The conditions that prompt termination of the treatment
3. The degree of confrontation of resistance

Time

The management of time (not only duration of treatment but also spacing of authorized sessions) in psychotherapy has taken on paramount significance in recent years and is an issue that many dynamically oriented clinicians feel ill-trained to manage. "Brief psychotherapy" can be as brief as a single session (Bloom,

1992) or as lengthy as 40 sessions (Malan, 1976), with the bulk accomplished in fewer than 25 sessions. The type of treatment may dictate the time frame, or rather (and less optimally) the time frame may dictate your choice of treatment. In either respect, it may be useful to consider distinguishing between the following three concepts, as outlined by Koss and Shiang (1994): "*threshold* (the lowest dose of therapy to produce a discernible effect), *potency* (the absolute amount of treatment needed to produce a specified effect), and *efficacy* (the maximum effect of a treatment when provided in its optimum dosage" (p. 669). *For better or worse, as psychodynamic clinicians most of us were trained to strive for efficacy, while managed care companies are satisfied with reaching threshold or potency. Thus, we tend to feel that externally imposed time limits necessarily compromise the treatment we provide.*

While the overall duration of treatment is of paramount concern to clinicians, managed care restrictions and the differing techniques of short-term treatment require us to reconsider the duration of the session itself (45- to 50-minute sessions versus a half-hour session or even 2-hour sessions), as well as the spacing of authorized treatment sessions (one session per week vs. biweekly or monthly meetings). Often, patients are preapproved for a fixed number of visits per year; thus, you or they may want to spread sessions out or engage in several brief courses of treatment over a longer developmental period. In addition, lengthening intervals between sessions actively discourages dependency and regression, an implicit condition for successful termination in many brief treatments. In short-term dynamic therapy, time can be more than a limiting and sometimes undesirable factor—it can be an overarching therapeutic factor.

Termination

Termination, in and of itself, is often a difficult process for both patient and therapist. In short-term treatment, especially in the context of managed care, termination is likely to be prompted by a number of factors other than the effective completion of a full course of dynamically oriented treatment. Termination is intrinsically related to, but not identical to, the issue of time. Termina-

tion is a process that varies depending upon the treatment strategy utilized, as well as the individual patient and his/her
psychopathology. The relative focus on the separation itself versus preventing symptom recurrence will vary according, in part,
to the transference orientation of the treatment, as will the
length of the termination process. This is independent of the
precise length of treatment. In some forms of brief dynamic
therapy, termination is a 3- or 4-session process that is clearly dic-
tated by the 12-session limit. Furthermore, the issue of separation is an explicit focus of the treatment. In other forms termination planned during the first session. Most of the approaches
allow for a somewhat flexible termination process.

Confrontation

In addition to the limitations imposed by often very specific patient selection criteria, therapists may shy away from certain
short-term dynamic psychotherapies because they necessitate an
active ego-confrontive stance that many psychodynamic clinicians are less comfortable with. The notion of confrontation is
also often misunderstood. It does not refer to the conventional
idea of assuming an aggressive, caustic stance with a patient.
Blamefulness is never helpful in a psychotherapy, and especially
in psychodynamic confrontation. What one is confronting, or
asking the patient to pay attention to, are dynamic structural
conflicts and inconsistencies in ego functioning, and their associated resistances. The discriminating feature of confrontation
in many short-term dynamic psychotherapies is the extent of un-
abated focus on the confrontational process. *Whereas in most psychotherapies one might not pursue a confrontative interpretive sequence
when significant anxiety is aroused, in certain short-term dynamic therapies this is precisely the point at which much learning is thought to
take place.*

CLINICAL EXAMPLE

In order to illustrate the use of some of the short-term therapy
variables identified above, as adapted to a more traditional psy-

chotherapy, consider the following vignette reported by Sperling and Lyons (1994, pp. 342–347). The case demonstrates how a transference-focused psychotherapy might have been used, but where a decision was made to approach the case from a short-term therapy paradigm without promoting therapist–patient transferential enactments, yet still examining and interpreting extratherapeutic transferences.

> This 40-year-old single woman presented with a childhood history of an alternately caring and physically abusive alcoholic father and an emotionally rejecting and often physically unavailable mother. Up until the time she presented for treatment, the patient's adult life had been characterized by avoidance and fear of emotionally intimate relationships. This manifested itself both in extreme social isolation and in an inability to take committed action that would lead to a stable and satisfying career. She came to treatment because of her perceived inability to make changes in her rigid and unsatisfying personal and professional life.
>
> It quickly became clear in treatment that although many transferential issues emerged, working directly with them was intolerable to this patient. She consistently refused to consider transferential implications of relational events, and she denied any but the most warm and affectionate feelings for the therapist. Any attempt to further examine some of the feelings that arose toward the therapist were rejected. Thus, for example, transferential interpretation of anger expressed not with words but with tone of voice, or analysis of projections such as immediately assuming, when a misunderstanding led the patient to show up 20 minutes late for the first session, that the therapist was very angry, were rejected. The patient steadfastly denied that any of her projections onto the therapist reflected anything but a consensual view of reality, apparent to all the world. Additionally, the patient initially expressed great relief in knowing of the time limitations on treatment and thanked the therapist profusely for telling her.
>
> Given what was known of this patient's past history and current functioning, events such as the ones described were taken as indications that for her it was important to maintain a perception of control over the setting and to clearly limit the dose of intimacy to be experienced with the therapist. The

question became how to work within these restrictions in a way that would lay the groundwork for their eventual modification while also facilitating a useful treatment outcome within the time period allotted for this treatment. It was clear that one could easily have spent much of the 7 months of treatment working with the patient's resistance to examining transferential elements within the therapeutic relationship, and particularly those elements relating to the patient's representations of attachment. However, it also seemed clear that given the patient's resistance to that kind of work, as well as the time limitations on treatment, this might accomplish very little. Therefore, a decision was made early on to put transference issues on a back burner. They were not ignored, however. The therapist tracked transference manifestations carefully, and used them for herself as markers of change and indicators of problematic representations. Transferential issues were occasionally introduced in sessions, in an attempt to test whether the patient could tolerate and work with them. However, they were not the prime focus of sessions; the focus with the patient became her functioning outside of the treatment situation.

Notwithstanding her vigilant defenses against awareness of the apparently considerable transference responses she experienced, the patient brought in rich material concerning her extratherapeutic interpersonal and intrapsychic experiences. In examining these experiences, she was able both to acknowledge patterns of relating to others and to see them as manifestations of enduring representations of attachment, as well as to gain some understanding of the genetic origins of these representations and of the ongoing and self-perpetuating influence they exerted on her processing of experience. In gradually understanding the origins and function of her need to control the dosage of intimacy in relationships, she came to recognize her characteristic style of nonaction, the self-protective function it served, and how it was maintained by the anticipation of negative outcomes in both interpersonal and professional situations. She was then able to see how taking any steps whose probable outcome was not easily expectable and controllable led her to quickly reject opportunities for intimacy and change. This process led eventually to understanding of how her need to control intimacy often resulted in her seeking intimacy with unavailable partners, and to connect these patterns with the recursive influence of enduring representations formed through her early attachment experiences. By the end of the 7-month treatment period, the patient was beginning to seek out and form more adaptive relationships, and was beginning to plan some changes in her professional life, the mere contemplation of which at the start of therapy had created unbearable levels of anxiety.

Cases such as this underscore the fact that some meaningful change can be engendered in an ego-supportive (and still ego confrontive and interpretive) psychodynamic psychotherapy within a relatively short period of time. The change usually takes the form of functional improvements, not the intrapsychic restructuring that might result from a long-term, transference-based treatment. *The bottom line here is that critical decisions about differential therapeutics can be made in psychodynamic psychotherapy, with interventions applied at a variety of dosages in order to achieve threshold or potency effects. That psychodynamic psychotherapy, like all other forms of treatment, requires such decisions to be made is a point lost on many managed care reviewers.* The fallacy still exists among many that dynamic psychotherapy is by definition always psychoanalysis or something very close to it. We all should work to dispel that notion.

7

Integrating Outcome Measures into Psychodynamic Practice

A majority of the psychodynamic treatment outcome literature (and a vast majority of outcome research in general) utilizes large groups of subjects to study treatment effects. Multiple-group designs with high numbers of subjects per cell allow researchers to make statistically sound conclusions, such as that the average subject receiving one treatment has benefited more or less than the average subject receiving an alternative treatment. This information is essential to verify the efficacy of psychodynamic treatment; however, it is of restricted utility in private practice. Managed care organizations don't want to know how the average patient responds to treatment, but rather how your patient is responding to the treatment you are prescribing. What becomes important, then, is to consider clinical in addition to statistical significance. This underscores the value of both single-group and single-case designs. The former examines differences among subjects in a group, all of whom receive the same treatment. No formal control or comparison group is included in the study. In the single-case design, which is usually the most practical for the clinician to implement in his or her private practice, the subject (patient) serves as his/her own control.

The typical objection to single-case designs arises from their restricted generalizability, even though, as Kazdin (1994) states, "most of the questions that guide treatment, as reflected in treatment evaluation strategies, can be addressed in the context of single case designs" (p. 31). Whether or not you have introduced formal outcome measures into your practice, it is likely that you are already using an informal intuitive variant of the single-case design to guide your treatment decisions. In making moment-to-moment treatment decisions, you have invariably made subjective evaluations of your patients' improvement (symptomatically or intrapsychically), as well as their need for continued treatment. In essence, managed care rewards (and sometimes requires) objective documentation of this subjective process.

Outcome research and psychodynamic practice are certainly not incompatible in the research literature and need not be considered incompatible in one's own practice. There are several clinically useful ways to integrate outcome assessment into practice, and doing so simultaneously offers a strong vehicle for supporting one's work with managed care companies. A commonly voiced objection to using the more standard outcome measures is that straightforward self-report measures of symptomatology do not necessarily measure the changes that occur in psychodynamic psychotherapy. Kazdin (1994) emphasizes the distinction between measures that assess change in symptomatology versus those that evaluate change in prosocial functioning, the latter referring to alterations that lead to more adaptive interpersonal relations. The two are certainly not mutually exclusive and at times appear to be unquestionably interrelated, but, as Kazdin (1994) asserts, "the overlap of symptom reduction and positive prosocial functioning may not be great" (p. 41). Traditionally, psychodynamic psychotherapy has been concerned with dynamic changes, reflected in interpersonal functioning, whereas behavioral techniques tend to focus on symptom reduction. This presents challenges for the psychodynamic therapist who must document "real" (i.e., symptomatic) changes in his/her patients occurring in a "timely" fashion. Structural and interpersonal changes usually occur less rapidly and are often difficult to quantify using measures that focus strictly on symptomatology. Thus, misgivings are warranted regarding some measures, and underscore the importance of choosing wisely and cautiously when picking outcome measures for your practice. With office use in mind, selected outcome research instruments that have demonstrated single-case meaning, particularly for psychodynamic psychotherapy, are discussed below, and their clinical use is illustrated.

The obvious convenience of self-report measures makes them particularly appealing to the researcher; however, for the clinician, particularly the dynamically oriented clinician, the following substantial cautions should be noted when you are choosing this type of measure for assessment. Critical questions are most often raised regarding the impact these measures have on psychotherapy. The pressure (if it is felt as such) to document progress may be perceived by the patient. It is not unlikely that the accuracy of these measures may be compromised by the patient's interest in pleasing you. As with other difficult issues that arise in psychotherapy, the treatment frame within which deviations are introduced is all-important. If you begin a treatment with the patient expecting that some outcome assessment will be a regular part of the process, it will likely be regarded as less of an intrusion; but to introduce it "out of the blue" in the middle of a treatment where there is no precedent for such material will understandably be regarded as an intrusion.

When self-report outcome measures are introduced at the time the treatment begins, they are typically perceived by the patient as a necessary adjunct to the diagnostic/assessment process. If presented as a tool to better enable the therapist to formulate a treatment plan and further guide the treatment, it has been our experience that patients rarely object. This is especially true if the patient understands that this information may increase the likelihood of reimbursement. Compliance is enhanced considerably by use of computer administration with adolescents (C. M. Grilo, personal communication, 1995), while at least one quality-of-life study of adults aged 17–81 suggested that pen-based electronic questionnaires were preferable to conventional paper-and-pencil administration, the former providing more complete data (Drummond, Ghosh, Furguson, Brackenridge, & Tiplady, 1995).

While the notion of providing specifics about the patient's therapeutic progress to a third party may violate our ideals regarding the preservation of confidentiality, these days most patients expect a certain amount of information to be shared with the third-party provider. Where information regarding progress in treatment will be shared with a third party, this of course should be communicated directly to the patient.

Although self-report measures are susceptible to response bias and/or falsification, managed care companies are increasingly relying on patient feedback to assess services provided by clinicians. There is also empirical evidence to suggest that the patient's perception of the treatment is more strongly related to outcome than some forms of "objective" assessment (Horvath & Symonds, 1991). Therefore, we will review a number of patient-report measures that are convenient in assessing symptomatic and structural changes, and also provide some discussion of clinician-rated instruments.

As previously discussed, it is vital to consider the underlying premise or theory on which a particular measure is developed. This is especially true for instruments that are founded on a hypothesis regarding a particular causal pathway of a psychological disturbance. For instance, the Beck Depression Inventory (BDI), apparently the most widely used measure of depressive symptomatology, is based on a cognitive theory of depression. Thus, although the BDI is sensitive to changes in depressive symptomatology that occur in dynamic treatment, the measure is slanted toward assessing changes in cognitive and vegetative symptoms of depression. The clinical sensitivity of an instrument, that is, its ability to detect the clinical phenomenon under study, may be dependent upon the type of treatment employed. This does not necessarily imply that a given measure cannot be useful, but rather that you should consider the theoretical underpinnings of any measure before integrating it into your assessment procedure.

There are a variety of domains in which therapeutic change can be evidenced. Below we present a sampling of measures organized around several categories: general symptomatology, specific symptomatology, personality (character) change, social adjustment, global functioning, intrapsychic change, and therapeutic/working alliance. We note in all cases the citation to the original or most important publication for each measure and, where relevant, note the name of the commercial test publishers (their addresses and phone numbers are included in Appendix B). While tests cost money when they are published commercially, this also usually makes them much more user friendly, and more often than not there are computer-scorable versions also available. Where a publisher is not mentioned, the test may be obtained either in the journal article cited or directly from the author (as noted in the journal article).

MEASURES OF GENERAL SYMPTOMATOLOGY

Symptom Checklist–90—Revised (SCL-90-R)

   Author: Derogatis (1975).
   Publisher: National Computer Systems, Inc.
   Clinical population: Patients aged 13 and older.
   Type of measure: Self-report.
   Time to administer: 15 minutes.
   Hand scoring: 11–15 minutes.
   Computer formats available: Computer administration, computer scoring, computer interpretation.
   Information provided: Three global indices of distress (depth or level of disorder, intensity of symptoms, and number of symptoms) and the following nine patient characteristics: somatization, obsessive–compulsive behaviors, interpersonal sensitivity, depression, anxiety, hostility, phobic anxiety, paranoid ideation, and psychoticism.
   The SCL-90-R is a self-report measure containing questions designed to assess symptoms of distress typically associated with psychopathology in outpatients. Patients are asked to rate each of 90 items on a 4-point Likert scale indicating the level of current distress.
   This measure has been widely used in treatment outcome research and has consistently demonstrated sensitivity to clinical changes. The SCL-90-R will accurately assess symptomatic changes that occur in dynamic psychotherapy and was used as an outcome measure in the National Institute of Mental Health (NIMH) treatment of depression outcome study; however, it is

primarily geared toward assessing behavioral symptomatology rather than other treatment effects. This is one of the better measures in terms of global assessment of symptoms, although it may be more useful as a screening tool to identify clinical complaints rather than to document symptom changes over time. Measures geared to the specific symptomatology that the patient is presenting (anxiety, depression, etc.) may be more useful for this latter task.

Brief Symptom Inventory (BSI)

Author: Derogatis (1993).
Publisher: National Computer Systems, Inc.
Clinical population: Patients aged 13 and up.
Type of measure: Self-report.
Time to administer: 10 minutes.
Hand scoring: 10 minutes.
Computer formats available: Computer administration, computer scoring, computer interpretation.
Information provided: The BSI is the short form of the SCL-90-R. Although the BSI only comprises 53 items, it yields the same nine scales as does the SCL-90-R. Adequate reliability and validity have been established in numerous studies (Derogatis & Melisaratos, 1983). Additionally, while the computer scoring on most measures requires you to send the form in to the publisher, National Computer Systems has a somewhat expensive but highly useful home computer scoring and interpretation package available for this measure.

MEASURES OF SPECIFIC SYMPTOMATOLOGY

Depression

Beck Depression Inventory (BDI)

Authors: Beck, Ward, Mendelson, Mock, and Erbaugh (1961).
Publisher: The Psychological Corporation.
Clinical population: Patients aged 17–80 (Children's Depression Inventory also available for children aged 6–17)

Type of measure: Self-report.

Time to administer: 5–10 minutes.

Hand scoring: 5–10 minutes.

Computer formats available: Computer administration, computer scoring, computer interpretation.

Information provided: The BDI is a self-report measure comprising 21 items, each of which presents four statements that differ in terms of the severity of a particular symptom or set of symptoms. For each of the 21 items, the patient is asked to mark the statement(s) that best describe the severity of the symptom(s) during the past week. The BDI yields a global score ranging from 0 to 63, indicating the severity of depressive symptomatology. Because of the brevity and clarity of the measure, individual items can also be utilized to examine the number of cognitive versus somatic symptoms the patient has endorsed.

The BDI is based on Beck's cognitive theory of depression. Despite this underlying theoretical influence, the BDI has been demonstrated to be effective in assessing changes in depressive symptomatology resulting from a variety of treatment approaches (cognitive, interpersonal, as well as dynamic psychotherapies). In fact, the BDI has become one of the most utilized instruments in documenting treatment efficacy for depression in outcome research studies.

The advantages of the BDI are readily apparent. It can be completed in minutes and can be administered multiple times with relatively little inconvenience to the patient or interference with the treatment. Furthermore, scoring is a simple and quick process, and interpretation is straight forward and clinically meaningful. In addition, because of its extensive use the BDI has established norms in differing psychiatric populations.

Equally obvious, however, is the main disadvantage of this measure. The face validity is so apparent that it is easily subject to unintentional response bias and/or intentional falsification. Furthermore, there is an overdetermined emphasis on somatic symptoms rather than on the interpersonal vicissitudes of depression. As a result, there has been some question whether items on the BDI are any more indicative of depression than the items on the Beck Anxiety Inventory (L. M. Hsu, personal communication, 1995). While the latter was designed to measure anxiety, it is also primarily composed of items assessing somatic symptoms. In fact, the argument has been made that self-report measures of depression and anxiety "do not measure discriminant mood constructs" and therefore should be considered "measures of general negative mood" (Feldman, 1993, p. 631). This, however, may be a limitation of the constructs underlying depression and anxiety (or etiological relation between the two disorders), rather than a reflection of some inadequacy of the measures themselves.

A more common complaint about the BDI is that its symptom content is not consonant with the DSM-IV criteria for depression. The Beck Depression Inventory–II (BDI–II; Beck, Steer, & Brown, 1996), the most recent revision of the BDI, addresses this shortcoming by including items that examine concentration difficulty, worthlessness, and loss of energy. In addition, while the BDI asks about symptoms experienced within the past week, the BDI-II requests information about symptoms within the past 2 weeks, which, again, makes it more consistent with the DSM-IV criteria for depression. The BDI-II has demonstrated content and convergeny validity in outpatient samples. Despite the aforementioned limitations of the BDI, it (and perhaps the BDI-II) is likely the most robust and easily administered measure of depressive symptoms.

Hamilton Rating Scale for Depression (HRSD)

Author: Hamilton (1960).
Clinical population: Adults.
Type of measure: Clinician rated.
Time to administer and hand score: 5–10 minutes.
Information provided: The HRSD is a clinician-rated scale of symptoms indicative of clinical depression. There are many versions available, ranging from 17 to 28 items (Grundy, Lunnen, Lambert, Ashton, & Tovey, 1994). The original HRSD, for which there is adequate reliability and validity established, has 17 scored items, with 4 supplementary items included for the purpose of evaluation.

The HRSD is mentioned here because it is probably the most frequently utilized clinician-rated measure (Williams,

1988). It is sensitive to clinical change and, in fact, tends to reflect greater treatment gains than the BDI or the Zung Self-Rating Scale (Lambert, Hatch, Kingston, & Edwards, 1986). Reasons for this finding are unclear and, as suggested by Lambert et al., may be a function of self-reported vs. clinician-reported means of assessment or, alternatively, the measures themselves may be assessing different facets of depression. This latter rationale also leads to one of the central limitations of the HRSD in assessing psychodynamic treatment gains: over half of the items assess behavioral and somatic sequelae of depression.

Depressive Experience Questionnaire (DEQ)

Authors: Blatt, D'Afflitti, and Quinlan (1979).

Clinical population: Adults (DEQ-A is available for assessment of adolescents).

Type of measure: Self-report.

Time to administer: 15 minutes.

Computer formats available: Computer administration, computer scoring.

Information provided: The DEQ is a 66-item self-report measure developed to assess differing subtypes of depression. It was developed based on an object relations theoretical approach. Subjects are asked to respond to items using a 7-point Likert scale ranging from strongly disagree (1) to strongly agree (7). Composite scores yield three factors: dependency, self-criticism, and efficacy. The measure was initially devised in order to empirically distinguish between anaclitic and introjective dimensions of depression. Typically, patients with anaclitic psychopathology are preoccupied with issues of relatedness such as intimacy, affection, and affiliation. These individuals are prone to depressive episodes resulting from perceived loss, separation, or abandonment. Patients who present with introjective psychopathology are more preoccupied with issues of self-definition such as achievement and autonomy. Thus, these individuals are prone to depressive episodes as a result of perceived failure or threats to their basic sense of self. Blatt, D'Afflitti, and Quinlan (1976) postulated that the items composing the dependency subscale were indicative of anaclitic depression whereas items loading on the self-criticism subscale were reflective of introjective depression.

Since its introduction, there have been some conflicting findings regarding the validity of this measure. For instance, results from one study suggest that "interpersonal dependency is more closely related to anxiety than depression" (Overholser & Freiheit, 1994, p. 71), whereas a second study indicates that dependency is, in fact, a "stable vulnerability [factor] to depression" (Franche & Dobson, 1992, p. 419). As noted above, principal components analysis of the DEQ has yielded three stable factors: dependency, self-criticism, and efficacy. Overall, there is evidence to support the test–retest reliability and construct validity of the dependency and self-criticism subscales of the DEQ.

The utility of this measure is that is purports to assess the construct of "depression" beyond behavioral symptoms. A recent factor analysis of the dependency subscale revealed two facets of this factor. The dependence component "appears to assess a generalized, undifferentiated dependence on others and feelings of helplessness and fears of desertion and abandonment," whereas the relatedness component "assesses interpersonal relatedness to particular significant, differentiated figures in relationship to whom there is a vulnerability to feelings of loneliness in response to loss and separation" (Blatt, Zohar, Quinlan, Zuroff, & Mongrain, 1995, p. 334). The former facet of the dependency scale is more highly correlated with both the BDI and Zung Self-Rating Depression Scale than is the relatedness component.

The utility of the distinction made above is that "it enables us to measure more precisely dysphoria associated with disruption in interpersonal relations . . . [as well as] . . . assess a more mature capacity for interpersonal relatedness" (Blatt, Zohar, et al., 1995, p. 334). Possibly as important is that there is evidence supporting the clinical utility of distinguishing patients with anaclitic versus introjective psychopathology (Blatt et al., 1988). Patients with introjective depression are likely to opt for more lethal methods of suicide, whereas patients whose depression is anaclitic in nature tend to make more nonlethal suicidal gestures (S. J. Blatt, personal communication, 1995). In a reanalysis of the NIMH treatment of depression outcome data, Blatt, Quinlan,

Pilkonis, and Shea (1995) found that patients who presented with introjective psychopathology were, in fact, less responsive to brief treatment interventions (whether interpersonal or cognitive-behavioral therapy). Discriminating patients by way of depressive subtypes using the DEQ may therefore be of significant relevance in determining an appropriate treatment plan (and, furthermore, justifying this plan). In addition, this measure may be more sensitive to a psychodynamic treatment approach, given its emphasis on character dynamics that are typically targeted in this form of psychotherapy. It is also amenable to multiple administrations in order to assess ongoing change during the course of psychotherapy.

Anxiety

Beck Anxiety Inventory (BAI)

Authors: Beck, Epstein, Brown, and Steer (1988).
Publisher: The Psychological Corporation.
Clinical population: Aged 17–80 (children's version is also available).
Type of measure: Self-report.
Time to administer: 5–10 minutes.
Time to score: 5–10 minutes.
Computer formats available: Computer administration, computer scoring, computer interpretation.
Information provided: The BAI is a 21-item self-report measure that assesses the severity of symptoms indicative of anxiety disorders. For each item, the patient is asked to indicate how much he/she has been bothered by a particular symptom during the past week on a scale from 0 (not at all) to 3 (severely). The BAI yields a global score ranging from 0 to 63, indicating the severity of anxiety the patient is experiencing. It thus enables the clinician to assess the physiological and cognitive symptoms of anxiety.

The BAI has advantages and disadvantages similar to those of the BDI. Briefly reiterated, the clear benefits of the BAI are ease of repeated administration and scoring, psychometric properties, and evidenced utility in documenting treatment changes. The primary weaknesses of this measure are the potential for response bias and/or falsification, and an overemphasis on somatic symptoms rather than intrapsychic phenomena.

One additional and significant limitation of the BAI is that it is an overall global measure of the very broad construct known as "anxiety." This measure does not effectively discriminate between different types of anxiety disorders, although mean scores for several diagnostic groups are available for comparison. Thus, it will provide an overall assessment of fluctuations in symptoms, but it will not provide more specific information useful for diagnostic and treatment decisions.

State–Trait Anxiety Inventory, Form Y (STAI-Y)

Author: Spielberger (1983).

Clinical population: Adults (children's version is also available).

Type of measure: Self-report.

Time to administer: 20 minutes.

Time to score: 10 minutes.

Computer formats available: Computer administration and computer scoring.

Information provided: The STAI-Y composes two 20-item scales that independently assess state and trait anxiety. For each item on the "state" form, the patient is asked to indicate how anxious he/she feels "at the moment." Each statement is rated on a scale from 1 (not at all) to 4 (very much so). Items on the "trait" scale are rated similarly, with the patient indicating how anxious he/she "generally" feels.

The STAI-Y is the most frequently used measure in evaluating outcome in anxiety research (Morin & Colecchi, 1995) and, since the introduction of the original version (STAI; Spielberger, Gorsuch, & Lushene, 1970), it has been used in more than 6,000 studies and translated into 48 languages and dialects (Spielberger, 1989; Spielberger, Ritterband, Sydeman, Reheiser, & Unger, 1995). Research studies and factor analyses conducted over the past three decades have reliably supported the state–trait distinction in evaluating qualitative aspects of anxiety (Cattell, 1966; Gaudry, Spielberger, & Vagg, 1975).

Briefly defined, *state anxiety* refers to transient episodes of unpleasant emotions characterized by "consciously perceived feelings of tension, apprehension, nervousness and worry, and associated activation . . . of the autonomic nervous system"; *trait anxiety* is understood as the relatively consistent propensity toward anxiety, which typically manifests as a proclivity to perceive a broader range of situations as potentially threatening (Spielberger et al., 1995).

Though the state–trait demarcation has been adequately validated, and the STAI-Y provides more discriminative information about a patient's anxiety than the BAI, specific treatment application of this information has been less well established. Nevertheless, the STAI-Y is an easily administered measure with sound psychometric properties that is useful in determining the precise nature of a patient's anxiety.

MEASURES OF PERSONALITY (CHARACTER) CHANGE

Minnesota Multiphasic Personality Inventory, Form 2 (MMPI-2)

Authors: Butcher, Dahlstrom, Graham, Tellegen, and Kaemmer (1989).

Publisher: National Computer Systems, Inc.

Clinical population: Adults (the MMPI-A is available for adolescents).

Type of measure: Self-report.

Time to administer: 75–90 minutes.

Hand scoring: 30–40 minutes.

Computer formats available: Computer administration, computer scoring, computer interpretation.

Information provided: The MMPI-II contains 576 true–false items, which combine to form 10 clinical and 4 validity scales that assess a broad array of psychopathology. The MMPI-II yields scores for the following 14 basic scales: lie, infrequency, defensiveness, cannot say, hypochondriasis, depression, conversion hysteria, psychopathic deviate, masculinity–femininity, paranoia, psychasthenia, schizophrenia, hypomania, and social introversion. While these clinical scales have names suggestive of diagnostic categories, they in fact are not isomorphic with diagnostic categories. The MMPI-2 is best interpreted as a profile, rather than examining individual scale scores.

For scoring of the scales, it is only necessary for the patient to complete the initial 370 items. The remaining items are comprised in scales primarily designed for research purposes; however, these supplementary scales can yield some useful clinical information. The clinician must determine, based on the referral question and presenting problem, whether the benefit of the information yielded by these scales outweighs the cost of asking the patient to complete the additional 206 items. While short forms of the original MMPI have been developed, there are currently none available for the MMPI-2 (Terranova, McGrath, & Pogge, 1993).

Millon Clinical Multiaxial Inventory, Form III (MCMI-III)

Author: Millon (1989).

Publisher: National Computer Systems, Inc.

Clinical population: Adults (the Millon Adolescent Personality Inventory and Millon Adolescent Clinical Inventory are also available for adolescents).

Type of measure: Self-report.

Time to administer: 30 minutes.

Hand scoring: 30 minutes.

Computer formats available: Computer administration, computer scoring, computer interpretation.

Information provided: A variant of its predecessors, the MCMI and MCMI-II, the MCMI-III consists of 175 true–false items, which combine to form 22 clinical and 3 validity scales designed to assess a wide range of psychopathology closely corresponding to DSM-IV diagnostic categories. The MCMI-III focuses on characterological/personality disorders (DSM axis II psychopathology) as well as symptoms indicative of clinical syndromes (DSM axis I psychopathology) (Craig, 1993). Information is provided for three validity scales (disclosure, desirability, and debasement), in addition to the following clinical scales: schizoid, avoidant, depressive, dependent, histrionic, narcissistic, antisocial, aggressive (sadistic), compulsive, passive–aggressive (negativistic), self-defeating, schizotypal, borderline, paranoid, anxiety, somatoform, bipolar–manic, dysthymia, alcohol dependence, drug dependence, posttraumatic stress disorder, thought disorder, major depression, and delusional disorder. The MCMI-III, while not as widely used as the MMPI-2, is a generally well-validated and popular instrument, especially in the assessment of character pathology.

Comparing the MMPI and MCMI

While these measures differ significantly in terms of the theoretical basis and underlying assumptions (or lack thereof) for test construction, they are discussed here together because there appear to be similar advantages and disadvantages associated with integrating these measures into your practice. Each of these measures is particularly useful for the purpose of differential diagnosis or strictly as a treatment outcome measure, but each is limited in its utility as a measure of ongoing progress in treatment. The MMPI-2 and to a lesser extent the MCMI-III are rather lengthy measures, which precludes multiple administrations without inconvenience (and irritation) on the part of patients. Furthermore, scoring either test is rather laborious if done by hand, although computer programs are available for both. Interpretation of the MCMI-III is slightly less complex than that of the MMPI-2 (given equal exposure and training); however, it becomes more difficult when you are examining configurations of elevated scales unless you are using a manual or computerized interpretation program. So-called cookbook interpretations are available for both. While neither the MCMI-III or the MMPI-2 may be the best choice to document treatment progress, they both can be quite useful to document symptomatic or characterological changes if administered solely at the beginning and end of treatment, or when you are attempting to establish your own database for factors correlated with treatment outcome. As previously discussed, it is always of significant value to be able to provide justification for the treatment which you provide, which includes documentation of the positive response likely from a given treatment with a given symptom or diagnostic picture.

Both the MCMI-III and MMPI-2 are useful—and recommended—for assessment purposes, particularly the former if you find that you are having some difficulty in making the differential diagnosis. While the focus of this chapter is assessment of psychotherapy outcomes, an accurate assessment of psychopathology is essential to treatment planning, and there is ample evidence to suggest that these measures can be of clinical value. Furthermore, with the number of allocated psychotherapy sessions limited, these measures may increase diagnostic reliability and expedite the diagnostic procedure so that more time is spent in actual treatment.

Personality Assessment Inventory (PAI)

Author: Morey (1991).
Publisher: Psychological Assessment Resources, Inc.
Clinical population: Adults.
Type of measure: Self-report.
Time to administer: 45–60 minutes.
Hand scoring: 15–20 minutes.
Computer formats available: Computer administration, computer scoring, computer interpretation.
Information provided: The PAI is an 344-item objective inventory that combines to form 11 clinical, 5 treatment, 4 validity, and 2 interpersonal scales. Ten of these scales (9 clinical and 1 treatment) are further divided into subscales designed to give more precise information regarding psychopathology. The PAI yields scores for each of the scales below, with subscales in parentheses.

Clinical Scales. Somatic complaints (conversion, somatization, health concerns); anxiety (cognitive, affective, physiological); anxiety-related disorders (obsessive–compulsive, phobias, traumatic stress); depression (cognitive, affective, physiological); mania (activity level, grandiosity, irritability); paranoia (resentment, hypervigilance, persecution); schizophrenia (psychotic experiences, social detachment, thought disorder); borderline features (affective instability, identity problems, negative relationships, self-harm); antisocial features (antisocial behaviors, egocentricity, stimulus seeking); alcohol problems; drug problems.

Treatment scales. Aggression (aggressive attitude, verbal aggression, physical aggression); suicidal ideation; stress; nonsupport; treatment rejection.

Validity scales. Inconsistency; infrequency; negative impression; positive impression.

Interpersonal scales. Dominance; warmth.

An exceptional feature of the PAI is its inclusion of subscales that help refine assessment beyond simple diagnostic criteria. For instance, the depression scale comprises three subscales (cognitive, affective, and physiological) that reflect the theoretical underpinnings of depressive symptomatology. This differentiation distinguishes the PAI from other measures and provides more specific and possibly more useful treatment information. This increase in diagnostic specificity may be particularly helpful in justifying a treatment strategy. This becomes more apparent when considering the subscales of the borderline features scale. The differing borderline constellations imply (and therefore may justify) different treatment interventions. While the MMPI-II does have supplementary scales to further refine interpretation, these subscales do not appear to be quite as clinically useful.

Recognizing the limitations of the dichotomous true–false forced selection procedure, subjects are asked to give responses on a 4-point Likert scale. Again, this distinguishing feature allows the PAI to capture more subtle variations between patients in terms of the degree of psychopathology. An additional asset of the PAI are the five treatment scales, which were "designed to provide information about potential complications in treatment that would not necessarily be apparent from diagnostic information" (Morey, 1991, p. 72).

The PAI has excellent reliability and validity, provides clinically meaningful information, and although administration time is equal to that of other broad personality measures, scoring and interpretation is significantly easier.

MEASURES OF SOCIAL ADJUSTMENT

Inventory of Interpersonal Problems (IIP)

Authors: Horowitz, Rosenberg, Bauer, Ureno, and Villasenor (1988); Alden, Wiggins, and Pincus (1990).

Clinical population: Adults.

Type of measure: Self-report.

Time to administer: 20–25 minutes (127-item version, Horowitz et al., 1988); 10–15 minutes (64-item version, Alden et al., 1990).

Time to score: 10–15 minutes.

Information provided: The IIP is a self-report instrument designed to measure interpersonal relatedness and associated distress. It consists of 127 items (64 items on the shorter, revised version) that are rated by the patient on a 5-point Likert scale. The measure describes different types of interpersonal problems and asks the patient to indicate how much distress each of these problems is currently causing.

This measure is particularly suitable for work with patients in psychodynamic psychotherapy for a number of reasons. First and foremost, this measure is focused on changes that are typically of interest to the dynamic clinician. Specifically, it taps into interpersonal difficulties that commonly are among the source of conflict for patients, difficulties which are often the central focus of dynamic work such as issues of control, assertiveness or intimacy. Furthermore, there exist empirical data suggesting that the IIP has sensitivity to clinical change in dynamically oriented psychotherapy beyond the change captured by symptom-oriented measures. Horowitz et al. (1988) demonstrated that while both the SCL-90-R and IIP were sensitive to clinical improvement during the first 10 sessions of treatment, only the IIP revealed change that occurred within the final 10 sessions in brief dynamic psychotherapy. This would seem particularly useful information for the dynamic clinician who must provide a managed care company with evidence of clinical gain in order to justify the need for and utility of additional treatment sessions. In addition, this measure can also be used to determine which patients might be able to benefit most from psychodynamic treatment.

Social Adjustment Scale (SAS)

Authors: Weissman and Bothwell (1976).

Clinical Population: Adults.

Type of measure: Self-report.

Time to administer: 15–20 minutes.

Time to score: 15 minutes.

Information provided: The SAS is a self-report measure that yields an overall adjustment score and scores for six specific areas of role functioning: work, social and leisure, relationships with extended family, and role as a spouse, parent, and member of the family unit. Within each area, questions are geared to assess "the patient's performance at expected tasks, the amount of friction with others, finer aspects of interpersonal relations, and inner feelings and satisfactions" (Weissman & Bothwell, 1976, p. 1112). Forty-two items are rated on a 5-point Likert-type scale.

In response to efforts aimed at early detection and prevention in the early 1970s, the SAS was developed specifically to identify asymptomatic individuals who exhibited social impairment. The prevailing zeitgeist at that time promoted early identification and intervention with an intent to preclude the development of more serious psychological difficulties. Thus, provision of services prior to the onset of symptoms was actively encouraged. The irony of this objective does not go unnoticed. The tide has shifted so dramatically that we are no longer able to provide treatment (i.e., with reimbursement) in the absence of symptomatic distress.

Interest in measures of social adjustment was also sparked by growing dissatisfaction with symptom scales as sole estimates of treatment effects. As with the IIP, the SAS has proven itself to be sensitive to clinical change beyond amelioration of symptoms and, similarly, changes in social adjustment manifested on this measure are expected to emerge some time after the reduction of symptoms. Again, ascertaining information about social adjustment appears to be crucial in the accurate assessment of the long-term efficacy of psychotherapeutic intervention.

MEASURES OF GLOBAL FUNCTIONING

Global functioning or quality of life measures are rapidly gaining favor with managed care companies. Although the primary limitation of these instruments is their lack of specificity, in their focus on subjective experience. This speaks to an issue of primary importance in dynamic work; people can be symptomatically "functional" or have objectively "intact" lives but still experience a high degree of psychic distress or inner turmoil that detracts from the overall quality of their lives. Moreover, measures of global assessment, particularly those that examine the vicissitudes of interpersonal relationships, appear to be more applicable within a dynamic framework.

Quality of Life Inventory (QOLI)

Author: Frisch (1994).
Publisher: National Computer Systems, Inc.
Clinical population: Adults.
Type of measure: Self-report.
Time of administration: 5 minutes.
Hand scoring: 10 minutes.
Computer formats available: Computer administration, computer scoring, and computer interpretation.
Information provided: The QOLI is a measure of general life satisfaction with norms based on responses from an adult nonpatient population. It yields one broad score measuring "overall quality of life," as well as subscale scores measuring the patient's overall satisfaction/dissatisfaction in the following 16 life areas: health; self-esteem; goals and values; money; work; play; learning; creativity; helping; love; friends; children; relatives; home; neighborhood; community. The QOLI can be used in assessment to determine goals for treatment and to identify areas of focus, and can also be administered to document ongoing progress resulting from treatment interventions. Given its easy home computer scoring and report capabilities, it may be of particular interest to clinicians among the measures of global functioning.

Short Form–36 Health Survey (SF-36)

Authors: Ware and Sherbourne (1992).
Clinical population: Adults.
Type of measure: Self-report.
Time to administer: 10–15 minutes.
Time to score: 5–10 minutes.

Information provided: The SF-36 is a multi-item scale that assesses the following eight dimensions of health: limitations in physical activity because of health problems; limitations in social activities because of physical or emotional problems; limitations in usual role activities because of physical health problems; limitations in usual role activities because of emotional problems; bodily pain; general mental health (psychological distress and well-being); vitality (energy and fatigue); general health perceptions.

The SF-36 was developed from an assessment measure used in the Medical Outcomes Study (MOS), a longitudinal study intended to explore patient, provider, and system of health care attributes that influence outcome in patients with physical and mental illness (McHorney, Ware, & Raczek, 1993). The SF-36 has become one of the more frequently used outcome measures in general health outcome studies and is likely to be widely recognized by managed care companies. Given its reference point of general physical, behavioral, and emotional functioning, as opposed to specifically mental health variables, it may not be the best choice if only one measure of global functioning is being chosen. As an adjunct to another functioning measure specific to mental health, it provides a useful broad health context.

Global Assessment Scale (GAS)

Authors: Endicott, Spitzer, Fleiss, and Cohen (1976).
Clinical population: Adults.
Type of measure: Clinician rated.
Time to administer/score (clinician's rating): 2 minutes.
Information provided: The GAS is a rating scale for assessing the general level of a patient's functioning, and changes in functioning, on a continuum from psychological sickness to psychological health over a period of time. Patients receive a single score between 1 and 90 based on their current functioning. The scale ranges from 1 (most marked psychopathology and compromised functioning) to 90 (healthiest functioning) and is anchored to descriptors at 10-point intervals, although a score may be given at any point on the continuum. The GAS score is similar to the Global Assessment of Functioning (GAF) rating given on axis V of the DSM-IV, except that the GAF is rated on a 1–100 scale.

The psychometric properties of this measure have been established in a number of studies, and furthermore the GAS has demonstrated a good sensitivity to therapeutic changes. Endicott et al. (1976) found that "the GAS ratings had greater sensitivity over time than did other ratings of overall severity or specific symptom dimensions" (p. 766). While this measure may appear superficially crude and is geared toward a behavioral assessment of the patient's functioning, pre-posttreatment change scores on the GAS have been found to correlate significantly with pre-posttreatment changes on a measure of quality of object representations (Blatt, Wiseman, Prince-Gibson, & Gatt, 1991). One caution to note with the GAS, however, is that the reliability (i.e., consistency) of scores across different raters (therapists) may be limited when they are without significant training and when consensual validity has not been established regarding the rating categories. For a single rater generating scores for a given patient across time or across many patients, the reliability of scores is much stronger.

Health–Sickness Rating Scale (HSRS)

Author: Luborsky (1962).
Clinical population: Adults.
Type of measure: Clinician rated.
Time to administer/score (clinician's rating): 5–10 minutes.
Information provided: The HSRS, which preceded the GAS, is a slightly more extensive version of it. In addition to providing a global scale, there are seven additional scales the clinician rates from 0 to 100: ability to function autonomously; seriousness of symptoms; degree of discomfort; effect on environment; utilization of abilities; quality of interpersonal relationships; breadth and depth of interests. The HSRS has been used extensively to measure treatment gains and outcome, and has established validity and reliability.

MEASURES OF INTRAPSYCHIC CHANGE

Proponents of dynamic therapy argue that techniques that challenge maladaptive defensive structures, interpret/confront maladaptive relational (attachment and object relational) patterns, and promote insight (often by attending to transference) are essential to therapeutic efficacy, particularly over an extended period of time. As a consequence of therapy, then, it is expected that these "process variables" will change as therapy advances. A commonly voiced objection to psychodynamic theory, and, by extension, psychodynamic psychotherapy, is that process variables are not measurable and therefore their utility (or even their existence) cannot be empirically validated. In response to the criticism levied at psychodynamic theory, researchers have attempted to identify, quantify, and measure these process variables. Specifically, relatively reliable measures of defenses, level of insight, attachment styles, quality of object relations, and therapeutic alliance have all been developed in the last two decades.

While these constructs are intuitively invaluable to the therapeutic process, their empirical validation is important for two reasons in the context of this discussion. First, the clinician can now provide empirical support that justifies the exploration of these variables in the treatment setting as valuable and warranted. Thus, for instance, we can now make a plausible (and empirically validated) argument that (1) "defenses underlie many psychopathological phenomena" (Perry, 1993, p. 274); (2) defenses are related to overall mental health and global functioning (Perry & Cooper, 1989); (3) defenses can be modified; and, by inference, (4) it is therapeutically useful to address intrapsychic phenomena such as defensive processes in therapy. A second benefit of empirical validation is that there is evidence to indicate that measurement of these process variables can not only provide useful information regarding outcome but can also measure ongoing progress in therapy. In our attempt to provide evidence of efficacy, utilizing measures sensitive to improvement in dynamic therapy is necessary. Thus, ongoing measurement of the therapeutic alliance, for example, can provide a valid indicator of the patient's progress in treatment (Frieswyk et al., 1986) and, furthermore, may help provide justification for specific treatment decisions. With that in mind, we will briefly present some of the instruments which are available to assess constructs that are central to a psychodynamic approach.

Defense Mechanisms/Styles

Defense Mechanisms Inventory (DMI)

Authors: Ihilevich and Gleser (1986).
Publisher: Psychological Assessment Resources, Inc.
Clinical population: Adults (adolescent version also available).
Type of measure: Self-report.
Time to administer: 30–40 minutes.
Time to score: 10 minutes.
Information provided: The DMI offers a method of categorization for the following five defensive responses to conflict: aggressive, projective, intellectualizing, intrapunitive, and repressive. Standardized scores (i.e., T scores) are yielded for each defense mechanism on four dimensions: actual behavior, fantasy behavior, thought, and affect.

The DMI presents patients with 10 vignettes and asks them to indicate how they would be most likely and least likely to respond to the situation described. Each vignette is followed by four questions with five choices corresponding to the five defenses measured: principalization, projection, reversal, turning against an object, and turning against self. The DMI is accompanied by a clinical manual that allows the clinician to determine which therapeutic interventions are recommended and which are contraindicated based on the patient's defensive constellation. Though this measure is not suggested as a reliable indicator of change in treatment, it may provide a method to justify specific interventions.

Object Relations and Mental Representations/ Transference

Object relations is perhaps the most clinically relevant concept to psychodynamic formulation and treatment, yet simultaneously the most difficult to measure. There are as yet no really strong *and* content-meaningful self-report tests available. The one we do present below is a step in the right direction, but this remains a fertile area for future research. There are several rich object relations measures available based on scoring of projective tests, yet the use of conventional projectives tests is, at present, difficult to justify in a managed care context. For a review of such measures, which may nonetheless be useful for the clinician's own formulation of a case, see Fishler, Sperling, and Carr (1990).

The associated concepts of transference and mental representations have been a more productive, albeit no less complicated, area of assessment. The majority of work in these areas too has evolved from the projective literature but has moved into some diversified methods. While these methods are as yet not crisp and easy enough in administration and scoring to warrant inclusion in a psychodynamic clinician's assessment battery (i.e., their administrations are time intensive, and their scoring requires much training), they are all quite rich and offer the promise of interesting clinical applications. For an interesting collection of papers on measuring transference-related phenomena, we recommend an issue of the journal *Psychotherapy Research* (Vol. 4, Nos. 3–4, fall/winter 1994) that applies seven transference-related measures to the same clinical interview data. The articles in this issue are coherent and effective illustrations of these methods.

Bell Object Relations Reality Testing Inventory (BORRTI)

Authors: Bell, Billington, and Becker (1986).
Publisher: Western Psychological Services.
Clinical population: Adults.
Type of measure: Self-report.
Time to administer: 15 minutes.
Hand scoring: 20–25 minutes.
Computer formats available: Computer scoring.
Information provided: The BORRTI consists of 90 true–false statements about the patient's "most recent experience." It yields scores for four object relations scales (alienation, insecure attachment, egocentricity, and social incompetence) and three reality testing scales (reality distortion, uncertainty of perception, and hallucinations and delusions). The manual for the BORRTI provides subscale descriptions, presents diagnostic implications for "high scorers" on each of the subscales, and further examines particular constellations of elevated subscales.

Norms are also provided to distinguish individuals with deficits in each of the aforementioned spheres.

While this measure has been used in several research studies, it has relatively less utility in a clinical context, as the scale content domains and scores generated don't offer as much clinical utility as many other measures. A positive feature is that it is normed on several clinical diagnostic samples.

Attachment

The concept of attachment offers a somewhat stronger array of measures in the self-report domain that are useful to the clinician (Sperling, Foelsch, & Grace, 1996). Since John Bowlby introduced the concept of attachment style and the notion of enduring internal working models (i.e., mental representations) of self and others, empirical research in this area has flourished. There is mounting evidence to suggest that attachment patterns endure over time and profoundly affect the quality of interpersonal relationships across the life span. We can expect, then, that the patient's attachment style will have implications for the therapeutic relationship and thus ramifications for intervention and outcome.

Hazan and Shaver's Attachment Self-Report (HS)

Authors: Hazan and Shaver (1987).
Clinical population: Adults.
Type of measure: Self-report.
Time to administer: 1 minute.
Time to score: No scoring necessary.
Information provided: Hazan and Shaver's (1987) attachment self-report consists of three brief paragraphs, theoretically designed using M. D. S. Ainsworth's tripartite attachment classification system. Patients are asked to indicate which of the statements most accurately reflects their feelings concerning intimate relationships, and their response yields an attachment classification as either secure, avoidant, or ambivalent.

As the first self-report measure of adult attachment style, this instrument has been utilized most frequently in the research literature. Because of its simplicity, however, it does not capture any subtle variations in attachment patterns. It is suggested as an overall indicator of a patient's typical attachment style, which could help you to conceptualize the kinds of transferential issues that are likely to emerge in the therapeutic process and thus have implications for the therapeutic alliance.

Attachment Style Inventory (ASI)

Authors: Sperling and Berman (1991).
Clinical population: Adults.
Type of measure: Self-report.
Time to administer: 10 minutes.
Time to score: 5 minutes.
Information provided: The ASI is an adult attachment style measure that differs from other measures of attachment in that it not only elicits information about the patient's "primary attachment style" in most relationships but also allows for the possibility that attachment styles differ between different categories of relationships. Thus, this measure provides information regarding the patient's primary attachment style within each of the following four relationship categories: mother, father, friendship, and sexual partner. It also yields a global score for each of the following four attachment styles: avoidant, dependent, hostile, and resistant–ambivalent. In addition, there is an item that measures overall felt security/insecurity across all relationships, as well as security/insecurity within each of these four relationships.

The ASI consists of brief descriptions of four attachment styles, as well as the aforementioned item that assesses a security/insecurity dimension. Patients indicate the extent to which each description applies to them on a 9-point Likert scale. The inventory is completed independently for each of the four relationships mentioned above. Ratings for each attachment style are collapsed across the four relationship categories to yield four global attachment scores. Several studies using this measure (e.g., Sack, Sperling, Fagen, & Foelsch, 1996; Sperling, Foelsch, & Grace, 1996) have supported its reliability and validity, and offer normative scores for general adult and character disorder samples.

MEASURES OF THERAPEUTIC/
WORKING ALLIANCE

Intuitively and theoretically, clinicians dating back to Sigmund Freud have known that the therapeutic alliance is central to an effective psychodynamic treatment. Within the past decade there has also been much empirical evidence to suggest that the therapeutic alliance is strongly and consistently related to various outcome measures (Frank & Gunderson, 1990; Hartley, 1985; Piper et al., 1991). A positive therapeutic alliance, as ascertained from both patient and therapist reports, has been consistently associated with successful therapeutic outcome as measured by social adjustment (Rounsaville et al., 1987), the Symptom Checklist–90 (Adler, 1988), the GAS (Bachelor, 1991), the MMPI (Moras & Strupp, 1982), drug use (Luborsky, McLellan, Woody, O'Brien, & Auerbach, 1985), and other measures. In fact, therapeutic alliance is proposed to be the strongest predictor of outcome in brief psychodynamic psychotherapy (Gaston, Marmar, Thompson, & Gallagher, 1988; Hartley, 1985). Moreover, therapeutic alliance has exerted an effect across a broad range of treatments including behavioral therapy (DeRubeis & Feeley, 1990), psychodynamic therapy (Luborsky & Auerbach, 1985), and cognitive therapy (Raue, Castunguay, & Goldfried, 1991).

California Psychotherapy Alliance Scale (CALPAS)

Authors: Marmar, Weiss, and Gaston (1989).
Clinical population: Adults.
Type of measure: Self-report and clinician rating (therapist and/or patient versions are available).
Time to administer: 10–15 minutes.
Time to score: 10 minutes.
Information provided: The CALPAS is a 31-item self-report measure comprising five subscales: patient working capacity, patient commitment, goal disagreement, therapist negative contribution, and therapist understanding and involvement. The CALPAS-P is the self-report measure completed by the patient, and the CALPAS-T is a similar measure completed by the thera-

pist. Patient and therapist respond to items using a 7-point Likert scale. The CALPAS is a widely used and well-established measure of therapeutic alliance in outcome research and can provide very useful information to the clinician. In light of managed care organizations' interest in patient response and satisfaction, it also offers a good tool in documenting treatment compliance and satisfaction.

In addition to the CALPAS, there are a variety of therapeutic alliance measures available to the clinician. Most are highly correlated with one another, although there are slight nuances that may make some more amenable to psychodynamic treatment. For instance, the Working Alliance Inventory is theoretically based on Bordin's (1979) model of therapeutic alliance, which is more focused on agreement on therapeutic tasks and goals than on the relationship aspect of the patient–therapist dyad. The CALPAS, however, is "influenced by both traditional psychodynamic concepts of the alliance and the subsequent work of Bordin" (Horvath & Luborsky, 1993, p. 565). Furthermore, in one comparison with the Working Alliance Inventory, the CALPAS was able to predict change across a somewhat broader range of outcome measures (Safran & Wallner, 1991).

SUMMARY

Prior to summarizing the issues raised in this chapter, we need to address one major area of omission. We made a conscious, deliberate choice not to include projective measures of assessment. Some may question our judgment in choosing to omit measures that clearly tap intrapsychic change, particularly the Rorschach test. This decision was based on the two guiding considerations of this chapter: (1) practicality and (2) clinical sensitivity. Simply stated, the Rorschach is a rich but time-consuming measure to administer, score, and interpret, and is not amenable to multiple administrations. Unfortunately, this is also true for many assessment measures with a foundation in psychoanalytic theory. Many of the reliable and valid procedures not mentioned in this chapter are excellent for establishing the efficacy of dynamic interventions in a research setting; however, they are not practical or time efficient in private practice. In addition, while there is a plethora of data to suggest that Rorschach variables are sensitive to psychodynamic treatment interventions, one is much less likely to be able to document these types of changes in short-term treatments.

At this point, after having been presented with a wide array of measures in this chapter, you may still be hesitant about introducing structured assessment into your practice, or you may be wondering whether most of the same assessment information could not be obtained as accurately, if not more so, by a trained clinician. The answer is, of course, yes. Much of the information yielded by the aforementioned instruments will surface in the therapeutic material as it unfolds throughout the course of treatment. This traditionally has been deemed the most effective way to gain meaningful clinical information from patients. Beyond the mere "facts" of clinical signs and symptoms, there are rich data to be found in the investigative process of disclosure; what the patient chooses to tell you, what the patient chooses not to share, and how long that process takes all provide the clinician with information beyond that of a self-report measure. In the days of long-term treatment this was the optimal approach; however, when you are faced with managed care organizations' constraints, your patient may benefit more from a relatively quicker assessment and treatment plan process, with more initial session time left to spend on forming an alliance and formulating treatment goals.

As we embark on an endeavor to negotiate with managed care, we should not forget that there are some treatment effects that will remain, to some extent, immeasurable. We cannot measure efficacy simply by looking at what has been gained but must also consider what has not been lost. In other words, a course of psychotherapy today may prevent the further development of psychopathology and the need for extensive psychotherapy (and therefore more cost) tomorrow. It is difficult, if not impossible, to measure what has not happened. Although community psychology has stressed the importance of prevention for three decades, managed care has all but dismissed the idea of therapy as a strategy of primary prevention. Patients must be in clear distress and conforming to the standards of medical necessity, and the nature of the necessity must be amenable to the type of treatment you are offering. Despite this stance, there are two realities we, as clinicians, should not allow managed care constraints to obscure. Beyond the immeasurable costs of pain and suffering, the fiscal costs of mental illness are staggering, and yet outpatient psychotherapy is a relatively small portion of these costs. For example, a whole year of once-per-week psychotherapy reimbursement will cost a managed care organization about the same as 2–3 days of inpatient hospitalization.

Beyond all of these considerations, we still believe that assessment always has offered and—even more so now—does offer an invaluable tool in every psychodynamic treatment. We have always practiced it implicitly and are being called upon currently to do so more often explicitly. You obviously cannot and should not incorporate all of the measures we have presented into your clinical practice, yet a careful selection of three to five measures at initial evaluation and two to three measures at regular follow-up intervals will offer both you and a managed care organization enormously valuable information. The exact choice of measures needs to be titrated to each individual case, although we do recommend at least one measure of general or specific symptomatology (chosen depending upon the patient's primary symptom cluster), one measure of social adjustment, one measure of global functioning, and one measure of intrapsychic change. From the material of this chapter, you should be well enough versed in the basics of outcome assessment to make reasonable choices and evaluate their utility for yourself.

8

Frequently Asked Questions and Future Trends

Having read and digested the material in this book, you may be left with considerable trepidation, wondering why you should even bother with managed care given the myriad potential problems. We want to emphasize that this book, especially in the early chapters, necessarily places exaggerated focus on negotiation of problems. While some of these problems may sound rather extreme, serious conflicts and patients who must be turned away are not an everyday occurrence.

Constraints on your work are another story. The remedies for these are hard to come by, but, as you have learned throughout, one of the main thrusts of this book has been the question of how a psychodynamic clinician can operate within managed care in spite of its serious limitations. *In practice, the majority of cases treated through managed care proceed rather smoothly, assuming that one learns to negotiate the constraints structured into a managed health care system and assuming that one is willing to tolerate the ethical and operational challenges. Managed care is far from an optimal system; it is still worth working with for many clinicians.* We have tried to present some useful guidelines to follow, recognizing at the same time that each patient, each therapist, and each managed care organization present a unique mix of needs and challenges.

PROBLEM SCENARIOS: CLINICIANS'
FREQUENTLY ASKED QUESTIONS

This section is intended to consolidate the discussion through-out the book by presenting several problem scenarios that psychodynamic clinicians may encounter in working with managed care. The material is offered in an FAQ (frequently asked questions) format. Although much of the material appears elsewhere in the earlier chapters, it is reframed here in a different fashion and designed to be readily accessible to the reader. The questions are listed in no particular order. We hope that it will be useful to have this reference of common questions to draw upon in "managing" your psychodynamic practice within managed care.

How can I write up a treatment review form to make it most likely that my patient will be approved for continued treatment? The keys are sticking with functional language and keeping it as simple as possible while still supplying all of the requested information. Secondarily, subtle mention of bad outcomes that might ensue were it not for continued treatment strengthens the argument. Overall, remember that if actually read, the report will be very unlikely to have more than a cursory reading, so get the essential points across succinctly.

If my patient is denied authorization for further treatment, how should I approach the managed care organization? Virtually every managed care plan has some appeal procedure in place, so the first step is to either check your provider manual or inquire of the company as to what the procedure is. If there is no formal procedure and/or you want to try to approach it more informally at first, ask to speak with a senior clinician reviewer. There is no guarantee that pursuing this angle with a more fully trained professional will yield results, but it may. Finally, you should inform the patient of the company's decision and suggest that he/she may wish to contact the company directly. Some managed care organizations will entertain such calls from patients, and some will only discuss treatment review decisions with providers; others can be swayed by patient calls. There is no magic bullet. It generally helps to know what the possible angles are and to use as many as are reasonable without becoming ineffective in your communications.

Can I treat patients who are covered by a managed care plan on a strictly self-pay basis if their benefits have run out for the year or they are denied further treatment? Going by the book, it depends on the stipulations in the provider agreement you signed with the managed care organization. Some specifically restrict you from providing service outside of the officially sanctioned process. Many others, including some of those that officially restrict it, will follow a "don't ask, don't tell" sensibility. If you deem that your patient has clinical need for further treatment, you have to balance your contractual obligation to the managed care organization with your professional and ethical obligations to the patient. You will need to decide for yourself.

Will new legislative efforts have any impact on psychotherapy under managed care? The brief answer is yes, but not in a direct way. Current legislative initiatives, including proposals for a federal patient bill of rights and other efforts in state legislatures to place controls on managed care, will help to curb the more flagrant abuses. The everyday assaults are unlikely to be legislated out of existence but are increasingly being held in check by the reality and perception of legal action. One thing is clear—loud and numerous voices are heard. Lobbying is an effective and necessary weapon, and professional organizations should be supported with time and money in their battles to regulate managed care.

How can I get on existing managed care panels as a preferred provider? When a panel is full, which most existing panels are, virtually the only chance of getting on it is if you offer something that not many others do and/or if you offer it in an area that is underserved. The something special can be a particular practice specialty, population, or spoken language. The geography just depends on the number of covered individuals for that managed care plan in their particular coverage areas. Whichever angle you pursue, it is probably wiser to market only one or two angles, rather than trying to present yourself as expert in 10 different things. This latter approach has less credibility, especially since the panel likely has providers with expertise in many of these areas already. Our experience is that clinicians who specialize in such areas as work with children and families, alcohol comorbidity, eating disorders, or specialized treatment protocols (e.g., dialectical behavior therapy, brief dynamic therapy, response prevention) will have the strongest argument for inclusion on a panel.

How much does managed care usually reimburse a therapist for a therapy session, and are all types of services and diagnoses covered? Managed care reimbursement levels have generally dropped somewhat in the past few years and seem to be at a stable point at the moment. The level of reimbursement can vary widely between managed care plans. Providers on HMO outpatient panels are almost always paid less than those on regular PPO panels, and in fact a managed care organization may have two contracts for different insurance plans, with two different reimbursement levels, with the same provider. Also as a rule, there is a differential rate paid to various mental health professionals by geography and terminal degree. Social workers are usually lower on the reimbursement scale than psychologists, who are lower than psychiatrists. In terms of services and diagnoses covered, virtually any DSM-IV Axis I diagnosis will be covered, although you need to be careful on reviews if you are treating in a specialized area in which you have little expertise. Some plans will cover Axis II diagnoses alone, but it is always wiser to include an Axis I as well, if appropriate. By far the most common service covered is the individual psychotherapy session, 45–50 minutes in duration, which has a CPT (current procedural terminology) code of 90806. Codes for shorter sessions lengths, for medical management, and for psychological testing are also available, but companies vary in terms of whether they will reimburse for these codes and, if so, how much. An important point to remember is that most plans will reimburse for one initial evaluation session at a higher rate. The CPT code for such an evaluation is 90801.

How do I deal with the stress of increased patient turnover? We wish there were an easy answer to this question. A reality is that given restrictions on the overall number of sessions for a course of treatment, if you work with managed care you will most likely have a higher turnover rate than otherwise. There are the obvious burdens this places on a clinician, like net increases in paperwork, but there are also hidden burdens, like the potential emotional strain of what can feel like incessant premature terminations. Perhaps the only adaptive stance to take on this issue, if one has already decided to work with managed care, is to ensure that you approach each treatment with full awareness of the likely restrictions and then let that guide the intensity and depth of the therapeutic relationship. There are many rewards from being helpful to a patient over a relatively short period of time, just as there are over the long term. For both the therapist and patient to be clear about the treatment limits ahead of time, and therefore about the available choice of interventions, is critical to emotionally "surviving," as well as offering sound treatment, under managed care.

Can I ever use the phrase "long-term treatment" when communicating to a managed care organization? Unless there is compelling reason to do so, the phrase long-term treatment should be erased from your communicational vocabulary with managed care. It is simply anathema to their way of doing business. When managed care patients need long-term treatment, it is best to present the work initially as moderate term, and keep justifying on subsequent communications why the targeted treatment closing date needs to extended.

On a treatment review, do I have to lie to gain authorization for long-term treatment of a patient in need? You don't have to lie, but you do often have to tolerate focusing on very selected aspects of your clinical work, and of course presenting them in a language that can be understood. In order to give the managed care reviewer enough reason to continually authorize treatment (within the bounds of the patient's insurance benefit limits), issues of medical necessity and deterioration should treatment be discontinued are the target. To achieve this will usually entail presentation of those symptoms and treatment events that enable you to emphasize pathology and prognostic challenge rather than adaptive functioning. However, there must also be some indication of positive treatment response in order to justify continued authorization. Negotiating this line between demonstrating need for treatment and demonstrating response to treatment can be difficult.

Will managed care eventually disappear and will things return to "normal"? Yes and no. It is very unlikely that we will see a return to the days of generous indemnity plans with bill submission and payment as the only interaction between clinician and insurer. What we may see more of over the coming years is less "management" of "routine" psychotherapies. This means that a preferred provider within a managed care organization who generally abides by the organization's treatment guidelines may be able to carry on with little management. We may also see a return of more unmanaged indemnity plans, albeit with less generous benefits for the patient and lesser reimbursement rates for clinicians. As the population ages and health care costs increase over the coming decades, there will be significant price pressures on the health insurance industry. We probably won't see providers shoulder a lot more cost reduction, as most of what can has already been wrung out of us. Someone will have to shoulder the increased costs, and this will preclude calmness and complacency in the health care industry.

How do I tell a good-enough managed care organization from a lousy one? The best indicator is the experience of fellow clinicians with that organization. So asking around is a first rank approach. This may not be so easy for many providers who have few clinician colleagues and/or few that work with managed care. State and local professional organizations are another excellent source of information. Most of them, if large enough, have some staff devoted to managed care issues. Further, there can be variation in practices within one managed care organization by region, so asking a local professional group about clinicians' experiences of that organization in that particular area is useful. Other factors to consider are the restrictiveness of the managed care organization's provider contract, the level of reimbursement offered, the parameters for treatment review (including simply the length of the review form), the number of providers already in your town or region (i.e., the greater the number of existing providers, the less are your chances of getting direct referrals), and the "mess up" factor. This last one refers to the uncanny ability of some organizations to "lose" treatment review requests and submitted bills, and the relative inefficiency of handling your phone calls and providing needed information. For example, simply finding out the benefit and copayment levels for a new patient can become an ordeal with certain companies, necessitating numerous phone calls and long wait periods, whereas for others one phone call with quick response will give you all the information you need. Anecdotal evidence and word of mouth are the most likely ways to gather this type of information, but it can't be underestimated as a pivotal factor in working with a managed care organization.

FUTURE TRENDS

As we stated at the outset, psychodynamics and managed care need not be completely incompatible, and there are trends in the managed care industry that might even promote some cautious optimism on the part of psychodynamic clinicians. Below we briefly address each of these trends separately:

Less Micromanagement

There appears to be a trend among some managed care organizations to apply less active management to the review of ongoing clinical cases. Whereas currently most ask their PPO clinicians to submit documentation for review at regular intervals, this practice may change in the years to come. Many managed care organizations are also developing what might be called "preferred" preferred providers. Such providers usually attain this status in one of two ways: (1) some clinicians will have submitted extra documentation to the managed care organization for specialty "credentialing," thus gaining the confidence of the managed care organization that they are especially qualified to treat certain forms of psychopathology within certain therapeutic modalities and will do so in a cost-effective manner; (2) other clinicians, by virtue of their track record in effectively treating patients covered by the managed care organization in a timely fashion, have gained the confidence of the organization that with minimal review they can conduct cost-effective treatments. On the one hand, this is certainly a desirable trend toward less micromanagement of cases, which is a time-intensive and nonreimbursed activity on the part of clinicians. On the other hand, the great worry is that, at one Machiavellian (but not too far-fetched) extreme, managed care organizations will reward only those clinicians that save the most money (i.e., conduct the shortest treatments) regardless of quality of treatment. This is a very worrisome prospect that demands strong advocacy from mental health professional and mental health consumer organizations. It is also one that might well become even more widespread were it not for potential moderating effect of three other current trends, reviewed below.

Focus on Quality of Care

If saving money was the mandate that had been practically deified by managed care organizations in their implementation over the past 10 years, the momentum is now beginning to shift in complicated ways, with signs of an impetus to move simultaneously in various directions (Noble, 1995). For instance, industry journals and newspaper reports have recently focused on a newly developing thrust for the next 10 years: quality of care. This may be fueled by an incarnation of the popular TQM (total quality management) movement of several years ago, or one of its recent reincarnations. This implies that in addition to controlling costs, employers, health insurers, and consumers are all realizing that saving money is not worth much if the quality of care stinks. This seemingly obvious realization is a welcome addition to the prevailing zeitgeist in the managed care industry, and we hope it will increasingly filter into the review and credentialing practices of managed care organizations.

Increased Responsiveness to Consumer Needs

Another related trend is an increased awareness of and responsiveness to consumer needs. After all, when employees complain enough about the overall quality and responsiveness of their health care organization, an employer may change its health insurer. This trend is manifesting itself in such things as increased surveying of patients' satisfaction with their psychotherapeutic treatment. Although this may be controversial to some therapists, we think that in balance it is a positive trend. What this practice means is that if you treat a patient under managed care review, after the treatment ends your patient may be sent a questionnaire assessing many outcome variables, including his/her satisfaction with your technique and responsiveness. Some psychotherapists object to this practice on ethical grounds (e.g., feeling that it violates the confidentiality of the therapeutic situation), and some object on substantive grounds (e.g., "I don't want quality of therapy to become a popularity contest"). Both objections have merit—more so the latter, since the confidentiality question is somewhat moot if you have already been working with and submitting reports to the managed care organization. The critical issue here is how managed care organizations use the satisfaction information. As with many forms of outcome/assessment data, to use it blindly as a full indicator of the quality of a treatment would be clinically unwise; to use it as a significant but not exclusive piece of information in evaluating the quality/outcome of treatment and the managed care organization's confidence in that therapist can be useful. In fact, it can provide one step in the direction of increased assessment of the quality of therapist practice postcredentialing, something which the field needs, given what seems to us to be the increasing number of therapists who practice outside of the bounds of reasonable technique.

Another trend toward increased responsiveness to consumer needs is reflected in the fuller range of plan options that insurers are offering. During the past decade it was quite common for an insurance company to offer only one, or at most two, plan options. For example, an HMO would offer subscribers the standard range of in-house services at reasonable cost, or another traditional insurer might offer either a major medical plan allowing for complete freedom of choice of providers, as one option, or a PPO plan, for somewhat lesser cost, as another option, where providers would be selected from an authorized panel.

The trend recently is toward offering a fuller range of options, perhaps four or five, all reflecting differing levels of care management, deductible payments, percent of services covered, and overall payment caps. This is an encouraging trend, as it represents consumers' demands that they have choice, and particularly that a point of service (POS) plan that allows for freedom to select any willing provider should exist. Of course, POS and traditional indemnity plans are always the most expensive options, but many do want to make use of them, and they have obvious advantages for mental health providers not affiliated with that particular insurer (i.e., they can still be reimbursed for their services).

Legislative Challenges and Patients' Bills of Rights

At both the national (congressional) and state legislative levels, there is a growing backlash movement to codify legal limitations on managed care practices. The push is to mandate systematic channels for appeals of treatment denial, provider disenrollment from panels, and refusal to pay for certain health care procedures. Recent national polls indicate that managed care is felt by a large majority of the population to be a problem in general, although somewhat paradoxically most people are also relatively satisfied with their particular plan. The conventional interpretation of such findings is that while most find their plans to be reasonable at the moment, there is great concern about the prospects for adequate coverage should their health care status change (i.e., worry that, if chronic illness or expensive acute illness develops, the insurer will not still fully authorize the needed treatment). The implication of all of this for the mental health community is that as managed care organizations feel politicians knocking at their doors, they may be more willing to self-police and modify some policies before they are legally mandated to do so.

Joining Provider Networks

If you are interested in working with managed care and are not already doing so, joining a preferred provider network would be one of the most common entry points. The trend however, is for there to be fewer opportunities in this direction. This is because the major provider panels are no longer in the start-up phase. It makes it harder to gain entry—but not impossible. A few pointers: be persistent; find an angle to market, such as a special treatment population or methodology; establish an office in a less well-served geographic area; find out when during the year the panel is reviewed, and apply at that time. Other tactics are to search for start-up managed care organizations that are just forming provider panels and are actively soliciting applications, and to apply to managed care organizations that have just gone through a merger, a point at which they usually reevaluate their provider panels.

These few ideas concerning joining PPOs represent an intentionally cursory discussion of an important strategic issue. If you do want to gain access to managed care provider panels, we suggest that you consult one of the several books that we review in the annotated bibliography in Appendix A. Many of these references address quite specifically the nuts and bolts of how to gain and maintain access to PPO networks.

Capitation and Independent Practice Associations

We discussed the issue of IPAs in Chapter Two, but it bears repeating as an important development in the fiscal and organizational provider structure for working with managed care. To review, an IPA is a group of providers who form a partnership and contract with managed care organizations to treat patients covered by that organization, often on a capitation basis. Capitation reflects a contractual agreement between the IPA and the managed care organization such that the IPA will treat any of a given group of "covered individuals" who present and are in need of treatment. Capitation agreements are appealing both to providers and managed care organizations because they guarantee payments and stabilize costs, respectively.

Aside from the question of the wisdom of such an arrangement, a more relevant question for the majority of psychodynamic clinicians, who are not currently in IPAs, is whether they should be joining one. To do so is no insignificant matter; it requires a considerable financial, time, and legal commitment. If you consider joining an IPA, it is best to be familiar ahead of time with your partners and to trust in their clinical competence. If you consider an IPA where you don't have a prior knowledge of the participants, try to investigate their credentials/reputations with local colleagues. This increased vigilance is called for, as being a partner in an IPA is a much more involved legal arrangement than, for example, being credentialed as an affiliated provider on a PPO or even doing affiliated treatment for (but not being a partner of) an IPA.

As to the question of whether you should join an IPA or not, this requires a careful assessment of the mental health care market in your region and, given this, whether you perceive that being in an IPA will enhance or diminish your ability to practice psychodynamic psychotherapy. Until a couple of years ago, our sense of the trend had been that providers not involved in an IPA would find themselves in a weak position vis-à-vis managed care organizations. We haven't, however, heard of widespread associations of providers into IPAs, so we now take a cautious stance and continue to watch for trends. There is obvious appeal for many of being an independent agent on a PPO, and others may thrive in an IPA organizational structure that explicitly supports psychodynamic work. It would be a nice outcome if the market eventually supported both types of provider arrangements—we'll see.

Uniform Billing

To a large extent uniform billing is already taking place, and it is likely to become the absolute standard for all insurance claims in the future. Uniform billing refers to the manner in which bills are submitted by a provider to either the patient or the insurance company. In previous years, virtually every therapist wrote bills by hand on his/her billing stationary and gave this bill to the patient, who then had the responsibility for submitting it to an insurance company if there was coverage. Increasingly therapists, especially those on PPO panels, are obliged to collect only the copayment from the patient and submit the bill directly to the insurance company for payment of the balance to the provider. Some companies will still accept handwritten bills on billing stationary, yet the clear trend is for clinicians to submit their bills on HCFA-1500 forms. HCFA stands for Health Care Financing Administration, which is an agency of the U.S. Department of Health and Human Services. The HCFA-1500 forms (12/90 revision) is the generic gold standard of insurance forms for any medical profession. Although this form may look confusing to someone who hasn't dealt with it before, insurance companies know exactly what to do with it. It contains basic demographic information on the patient, such as name, address, social security number, insurance company, and provider information, as well as CPT (current procedural terminology) code(s), diagnostic code(s), and fee(s) charged.

HCFA-1500 forms may be obtained in large quantities from several sources, including the American Medical Association. For most therapists, small quantities are all that is needed, and there are surprisingly few sources for this. One such source that we have had good experience with is a company called CWIB (Concerned Women in Business [800-233-2942]).

A considerable aid in billing in general, and especially in generating HCFA billing, are the several available computer software programs that do this task. One that we like especially is called Therapist Helper (Brand Software [800-343-5737]). This program does all sorts of billing, and additionally can take on most of your charting functions, with record of session dates/ fees, clinical notes, and a variety of background information. Therapist Helper comes in a full-use version (a virtually unlimited number of patients can be entered), as all the available programs do, but it also comes in a starter version for those who have a part-time practice. This version costs much less because it is programmed to handle a maximum of 12 patient records at any time, but it still offers the full range of functions as the full-use version. The integration of computer technology into psychotherapy practices, for billing, record keeping, and assessment purposes, will continue to grow. After an initial start-up period in which the learning curve is steep and using computer technology may actually consume much more time than otherwise, it can make certain tasks much easier. For insurance billing especially it is enormously useful.

An even newer and relatively unused (by private practice clinicians) form of insurance billing is electronic submission. With this form of billing there is no paper generated, only an initial signature from the patient authorizing you to share information with the relevant insurance company and to bill and be paid for your services directly. Electronic billing is more relevant for physicians or other providers who do a large volume of billing with particular insurance companies, but it is worth looking into if in your practice you work frequently with a particular company. In addition to obviating the need to generate paper, electronic submission typically results in receiving payment more quickly. Many insurance companies, especially Medicare and the Blue Cross/Blue Shield systems, like electronic submission, and if you have a computer with a modem and do some volume with these companies, it may be of interest.

So now, as a practicing clinician, and after having read eight chapters of material on psychodynamics and managed care, are you any more informed about managed care than you were before you began this book? Do you feel interested in working with managed care? Do you feel better able to advocate against areas of mismanagement by managed care? Do you feel that the only responsible stance for a psychodynamic clinician is outright rejection of managed care? To the first question of being better informed, we hope that your answer is an unequivocal yes. To the other three questions, each therapists's answer may be different. Whatever approach you take, we hope that you have found this book useful and that you reach decisions regarding managed care that work for you and your patients.

It shouldn't be any mystery by this point that we believe that some accommodation to managed care can be effected responsibly, but it is not the only reasonable stance for a psychodynamic clinician. Many still choose to reject managed care, feeling that it represents an irreparable violation of psychodynamic principles and ethical practice. Others devote their energy to advocating against managed care organizations for better patient and provider conditions. Still others work through the legal and legislative systems to contain managed care. If one chooses to work at all with managed care, we view the need for advocacy as paramount. Managed care is not a static construction—it has changed and will continue to change over the years to come. The point of advocacy leverage is that managed care organizations respond to market forces, lobbying pressures, and a developing wave of wrongful treatment liability lawsuits. Through the systematic efforts of professional organizations and, even better, organized patient lobbying efforts, psychodynamics can have a positive influence on the course of managed care. Psychodynamics and managed care need not represent an absolute oxymoron, just a relative one.

APPENDIX A

Annotated Bibliography of Managed Care Resource Books for Clinicians

There are a lot of books for clinicians on general managed care strategies that have nothing to do with psychodynamics and say essentially the same thing. Roughly 75% of the books on managed care cover a similar range of topics, and for that reason we have not included many in this annotated bibliography that may be well written but whose content is not sufficiently dissimilar, or whose material is somewhat dated such that they don't offer anything new to the clinician. We have included a few recent general reference works that offer managed care overviews and specific strategies, as well as several books that address a unique angle for psychodyanamic clinicians in the managed care arena.

Browning, C. H., & Browning, B. J. (1996). *How to partner with managed care: A "do-it-yourself kit" for building working relationships and getting steady referrals*. New York: Wiley.

This useful book is about as "nuts and bolts" as it gets; it is filled with 1–3 page treatments of just about every pragmatic topic there is of relevance to mental health care providers. To some it will represent a wealth of the type of valuable, hands-on managed care information they are hungry for; to others it will represent their worst nightmare of mental health care as pragmatic strategy devoid of any stable theoretical base or value system; to us it represents both.

Davis, J. (Ed.). (1996). *Marketing for therapists: A handbook for success in managed care*. San Francisco: Jossey-Bass.

The key word here is marketing, and this is clearly this book's strong and only suit. In various well-written chapters it systematically addresses how a behavioral health provider can successfully market his/her practice in a managed care context. About half of the book discusses every aspect of how to find, get access to, and maintain active status in a preferred provider panel, and the balance discusses other relevant marketing issues, such as "customer" service and promoting your services. While marketing is anathema to most clinicians, managed care makes it a necessary reality, especially for those who can't rely completely on word-of-mouth and existing peer networks for referrals.

Kaley, H., Eagle, M. N., & Wolitzky, D. L. (Eds.). (1999). *Psychoanalytic therapy as health care: Effectiveness and economics in the 21st century*. Hillsdale, NJ: Analytic Press.

This is the only other book we know of that directly addresses psychodynamics and managed care. The perspective in this edited volume is clearly that managed care has succumbed to quick fixes and thus has overlooked many of the benefits to be gained from intensive (i.e., psychoanalytic) psychotherapy for a range of disorders. As with many edited books, the chapters are variable in their quality and usefulness, yet there is much here that will be read as comforting and helpful to any dynamic clinician. This is, however, much more of a conceptual than a "how to" book. Many chapters discuss the politics and history of—and prospects for—psychodynamics within managed care, and this alone is worth the price of admission.

MacKenzie, K. R. (Ed.). (1995). *Effective use of group therapy in managed care*. Washington, DC: American Psychiatric Press.

For those who use group therapy methods in their clinical work, or those who would like to learn more about group therapy, this edited book can be useful. Its focus on the application of group therapy in managed care settings is unique and should be of much interest to specialized audiences. As group therapy offers a cost-effective and clinically effective form of treatment that is appealing to managed care organizations, more psychodynamic clinicians would be wise to become versed in these methods if they practice or want to refocus their practice in a setting where group treatment is practicable. Another appeal of this book is that several of its chapters emphasize psychodynamic group approaches and give specific examples of how to conduct such treatments consistent with managed care principles.

Poynter, W. L. (1998). *The textbook of behavioral managed care: From concept through management to treatment.* Bristol, PA: Brunner/Mazel.

This new book by William L. Poynter is less easily readable than his earlier one, but it does something most others don't; it is loaded with sample forms. These forms include such things as intake, treatment review, mental status assessment, symptom indices, and consent forms. The book is packed with information, often too packed for comfortable reading, but—as a textbook should—it offers an excellent reference guide. There is systematic attention to every aspect of case management under managed care, albeit from a theoretically neutral and bland stance.

Shueman, S. A., Troy W. G., & Mayhugh, S. L. (Eds.). (1994). *Managed behavioral health care: An industry perspective.* Springfield, IL: Thomas.

The table of contents of this edited book doesn't distinguish it greatly from a host of other managed care books. What does distinguish it and makes it useful reading are the authors, who are all top administrators in managed care practices or organizations, yet who are also largely clinicians. This view from inside the managed care system by clinicians, while a bit dated by now, still offers some new and interesting perspectives.

Tuttle, G. M., & Woods, D. R. (1997). *The managed care answer book for mental health professionals.* Bristol, PA: Brunner/Mazel.

This book covers familiar general ground in behavioral managed care, but it does so in a unique question-and-answer format, with emphasis on negotiation of pragmatic practice issues. For this reason alone, as well as its well-written and conceived narrative, we recommend it. This format is more easily accessible for many readers.

Zieman, G. L. (1998). *Handbook of managed behavioral healthcare: A complete and up-to-date guide for students and practitioners.* San Francisco: Jossey-Bass.

This book, like many others, covers the basics of managed care practice. What we like here is that the narrative is a bit more coherent and there is good attention to helping the clinician develop a real understanding of the foundations of managed care, before getting directly to the "how to." The field is crowded with generalist managed care books such as this, yet this would be one of our front-of-the-pack picks for such topic coverage.

There are three additional books that we include not because they discuss managed care issues per se but because they present material that is directly useful to one's clinical practice in a managed care environment.

Bernstein, B. E., & Hartsell, T. L. (1998). *The portable lawyer for mental health professionals: An A–Z guide to protecting your clients, your practice, and yourself.* New York: Wiley.

This is a book that every clinician should have on his/her shelf. The reasons should be self-evident. The world at large is increasingly litigious, and managed care exacerbates the potential hazards for clinicians. Being unaware is not an effective defense.

Jongsma, A. E., Jr., & Peterson, L. M. (1995). *The complete psychotherapy treatment planner.* New York: Wiley.

An investment in this book will save a clinician lots of time and energy while he/she is writing up treatment reports for managed care organizations. For 34 different symptom clusters/presenting problems, the authors systematically and briefly list behavioral definitions, long-term treatment goals, short-term objectives, common therapeutic interventions, and diagnostic suggestions. It is a succinct, easy to follow, and eminently sensible reference guide to treatment planning. Although there is always a danger of "cookbook" treatment approaches being used by those not well schooled in theories of psychotherapy, when approached by a well-informed reader this book can become an invaluable companion. We recommend it strongly, as well as two other recent book of similar form by the first author—one addressing child and adolescent treatment planning; the other, couples therapy treatment planning.

Zuckerman, E. L. (1995). *Clinician's thesaurus: The guidebook for writing psychological reports* (4th ed.). New York: Guilford Press.

This book is packed, almost too packed, with valuable information. Its focus is broader than that of the book above, and its style is more dense. This reference work offers suggestions on all aspects of mental health report writing, not just treatment planning. As the name implies, it contains a thesaurus-like iteration of terminological/conceptual possibilities in generating reports. Becoming familiar enough with the rather confusing structure of the book takes a little time but is ultimately worth it for the wealth of information provided. (*Note:* This book is one in a series called The Clinician's Toolbox, a Guilford imprint, which also includes another useful work entitled *The Paper Office.*)

APPENDIX B

Commercial Test, Supply, and Software Publishers Cited in This Book

Brand Software
Phone: 800-343-5737
Fax: 781-937-3232
Address: 500 West Cummings Park, Suite 1950, Woburn, MA 01801
WebSite: http://www.helper.com

Concerned Women in Business (CWIB)
Phone: 800-233-2942
Fax: 630-257-8418
Address: 358 Keepatau Drive, Lemont, IL 60439

National Computer Systems, Inc. (NCS)
Phone: 800-627-7271 (8 A.M.–6 P.M. [CST], M–F)
Fax: 800-632-9011 (24 hours/day)
Address: NCS Assessments, P.O. Box 1416, Minneapolis, MN 55440
WebSite: http://www.ncs.com

Psychological Assessment Resources, Inc. (PAR)
Phone: 800-331-TEST (8378) (8 A.M.–8 P.M. [EST], M–F)
Fax: 800-727-9329 (24 hours/day)
Address: PAR, Inc., P.O. Box 998, Odessa, FL 33556
WebSite: http://www.parinc.com

The Psychological Corporation (PsychCorp)
Phone: 800-211-8378 (7 A.M.–7 P.M. [CST], M–F)
Fax: 800-232-1223
Address: The Psychological Corporation, P.O. Box 839954,
San Antonio, TX 78283-3954
WebSite: http://www.hbem.com

Western Psychological Services (WPS)
Phone: 800-648-8857 (7:30 A.M.–4:30 P.M. [PST], M–F)
Fax: 310-478-7838
Address: WPS, 12031 Wilshire Boulevard, Los Angeles, CA 90025-1251
WebSite: http://www.wpspublish.com

APPENDIX C

Glossary of Health Care and Health Insurance Terms

Acute care: Medical care for illness or injury, typically with severe symptoms that emerge quickly, such as an accident, appendicitis, or heart attack.

Administrative costs: Costs related to overhead rather than to patient care, such as billing, marketing, claims processing, support services, and general management costs.

Admission: An overnight confinement to a hospital or other facility.

Adverse selection: The natural inclination for individuals to seek out lower premiums, which may not adequately reflect the risk associated with their medical condition; also the inclination of individuals with poor health, or expectation of poor health, to continue insurance coverage when healthier individuals may not.

An insurance plan suffers from adverse selection when it ends up with a disproportionate number of high risk individuals in its plan who have the potential to drive up claims, possibly threatening the long-term solvency of the plan. The plan may have to raise premiums to compensate, thus driving off the healthier individuals and further exacerbating its financial predicament.

Ambulatory services: Services that are rendered when the patient is not confined overnight. Ambulatory/outpatient services include, but are not limited to, the following: ambulatory surgery, office visits, home visits, outpatient services, and emergency room services.

Ancillary services: Medical services, such as laboratory and radiology, associated with an admission to a hospital or other medical facility.

Annual out-of-pocket maximum: Under an insurance policy, the maximum amount the insured individual will have to pay for covered services. Most covered expenses in excess of this limit will be paid by the insurer. The maximum may or may not include the deductible.

Assignment of benefits: The signed transfer of benefits of a policy by the owner of the policy to a third party, such as a physician or other service provider.

Balance billing: The act of billing the patient for the balance after the insurance carrier has paid its share, when the cost of the provider's services exceed what the insurance carrier will pay.

Beneficiary: The person(s) that a particular health plan covers.

Capitation: A payment method used by HMOs where providers are paid a prenegotiated annual fixed fee per patient regardless of the services that patient uses. In theory, this discourages delivery of unnecessary medical services.

Carryover deductible: A policy provision that allows covered expenses incurred in the last 3 months of the calendar year to be carried over to the new year and counted toward satisfying the new year's deductible. Avoids the hardship of having to meet the deductible at the end of one year and then again at the beginning of the next year.

Case management: A management process whereby a patient's care is closely monitored by a health professional. For example, a hospital or an insurance company may assign a case manager who is responsible for determining how many and what services are needed, as well as when certain services can be used (e.g., whether a specialist should be seen, whether the patient should go to the

hospital, or how long a hospital stay is required). Some health insurance companies use case management for patients who require
very expensive, intensive treatment for conditions such as heart
disease, cancer, and AIDS.

Catastrophic care: Life-threatening conditions that are expensive to
treat, such as organ transplants.

Certificate of need: A health care cost-containment strategy, mostly
used by states to require that health care providers obtain prior
approval of a government agency and provide proof that an expensive piece of equipment or facility is needed.

Chronic care: Care for long-term illnesses, such as nursing home care.

Closed panel: *See* Managed care.

COBRA (Consolidated Omnibus Budget Reconciliation Act): A 1986
federal law that mandates that terminating employees (and their
spouses and certain dependents, where applicable) must be offered the opportunity to purchase continued coverage under the
group's health plan for a limited period of time. The law affects all
public and private employers with more than 20 employees who
offer health benefits. The employer is allowed to charge an administrative fee in addition to the cost of coverage.

Coinsurance: Under an insurance policy, the percentage of the bill
that the individual must pay out of pocket, after the deductible is
met. For example, an 80/20 policy would mean that the insurance
company pays 80% and the individual is responsible for the remaining 20%. Not to be confused with copayments (*see below*).

Community rating: An insurance rating practice where the carrier establishes premium rates that cover a broad area, such as a geographic region, rather than basing them on the risks associated
with each discrete segment of the community, such as an individual employer or other type of group with insurance coverage.

Comprehensive plan: A type of indemnity insurance policy that covers
both hospitalization and major medical. Reimbursement is subject
to a single annual deductible and coinsurance for covered expenses
under both the hospitalization and major-medical portions.

Concurrent review: An ongoing review by a third party of the medical necessity, level of care, length of stay, appropriateness of services, and discharge planning for an inpatient hospital stay, conducted simultaneously to the patient's treatment.

Continuity of coverage: *See* Insurance reform.

Conversion privilege: A provision in a group health policy that allows conversion to an individual policy without providing evidence of insurability if the group coverage is terminated.

Coordination of benefits: A provision in most health insurance policies that addresses patients covered by more than one policy (e.g., a spouse's plan). In such cases the benefits are coordinated with any other plan's benefits so the patient may receive reimbursement up to 100% of the medical expenses covered.

Copayment: A form of cost sharing that requires the patient to pay a fixed fee toward the cost of each service used. For example, a prescription drug benefit may require a copayment of $5 per prescription, regardless of the cost of the medication. A copayment is a fixed fee and not a fixed percentage (as with coinsurance).

Cost containment: Any activity an employer, health insurance company, or health care provider undertakes to help keep health care costs from rising. Such activities might include preadmission certification, concurrent review, and case management.

Cost sharing: The cost that the patient incurs as a result of his/her care due to the insurance policy deductible, copayment, or coinsurance.

Cost shifting: Action taken by medical providers to recover revenue lost because of uncompensated care or undercompensated care that the provider has delivered. These costs typically are passed on to other individuals and private insurance plans in the form of higher prices.

Covered expenses: Hospital, medical, and miscellaneous health care expenses incurred by the patient that entitle him/her to a payment of benefits under a health insurance policy.

Deductible: The annual threshold of out-of-pocket expenses that an individual must incur before insurance coverage begins. For example, a $250 deductible means that an individual is responsible for the first $250 of expense annually before the insurance company begins to pay.

Dependent coverage: Health insurance that extends coverage to the legal dependents of an employee, usually a spouse, minor children, and/or elderly parents. Also known as family coverage. The definition may vary from one insurer to another.

Diagnosis-related grouping (DRG) system: A system used by Medicare to categorize all medical diagnoses under 478 groupings, with fixed reimbursement rates for each category regardless of the cost incurred. Providers, in this case usually hospitals, keep the difference when actual costs for a patient's treatment fall below the reimbursement rate; they incur the loss when actual costs are above the reimbursement rate.

Discharge planning: The process of ensuring that patients are discharged from a hospital as soon as medically appropriate, with planned, appropriate follow-up care as needed.

Effective date: Under a health insurance policy, the date on which the coverage begins.

Eligibility date: The date on which an individual member of a specified group becomes eligible to apply for health insurance under a benefits plan.

Employee Retirement Income Security Act (ERISA): A federal law passed in 1974 that was designed to set standards and protect the integrity of employee welfare and pension plans. ERISA has had unanticipated consequences for state health care reform efforts because it preempts some state actions. For example, it limits the ability of states to tax or regulate self-insured employee health benefits plans.

Employer mandate: A provision included in health care reform legislation that requires that employers provide and/or pay for employee health benefits.

Entitlement: Government programs under which citizens are entitled benefits because they meet certain criteria, such as age or poverty status. Examples include Social Security, Medicare, and Medicaid.

Exclusion or exceptions: Under an insurance policy, medical conditions or circumstances that are not covered. These may be an illness, such as a preexisting condition, or a type of care, such as office visits, that are not included in the coverage.

Exclusive provider organization (EPO): A type of insurance coverage that seeks to provide services exclusively through a particular network of providers. Typically services of a nonemergency nature provided outside the network are not covered.

Experience rating: An insurance rating practice wherein the carrier establishes premium rates based on the claims experience of that particular insured group such as an individual employer.

Fee-for-service method: A method of reimbursing health care providers based on the fees charged by the provider for each of the services rendered. *Compare to* Capitation *and* Fee schedule.

Fee schedule: A method of reimbursing health care providers that uses a list of maximum allowable fees for specific services and procedures. *Compare to* Fee-for-service method *and* Capitation.

First dollar coverage: A type of coverage in which medical expenses are paid by a health insurance plan without use of deductibles, copayments, or coinsurance.

Flexible benefit plan: An employer-provided benefit plan that allows employees to choose among a variety of benefits options and benefit levels.

Flexible spending account: An employer-provided benefit plan organized under Section 125 of the Internal Revenue Code. These accounts allow the employer to hold employee funds as well as employer contributions in an account from which the employee can be reimbursed far a variety of expenses, such as day care and medical expenses. The employee reimbursements, subject to limits, are not subject to federal income tax.

Gatekeeper physician: A primary care provider responsible for managing medical treatment of a patient enrolled in a health plan.

Guaranteed issue: *See* Insurance reform.

Guaranteed renewal: *See* Insurance reform.

Health alliance: Usually refers to a purchasing cooperative (especially those proposed under federal health care reform efforts) that negotiates health plans on behalf of its members.

Health benefits (health care benefits or benefits): Payments made by a third party, such as an insurance company, that cover all or part of the medical costs of a patient.

Health Care Financing Administration (HCFA): A division of the U.S. Department of Health and Human Services. It administers both of the major public health insurance programs: (1) Medicare, which covers people age 65 and older, and (2) Medicaid, which covers the poor.

Health care reform: Legislative attempts at the federal or state level to address a broad range of issues pertaining to the delivery and financing of health care. These reforms may involve changes in the regulation of health insurance, but typically they include other factors involved in the cost and delivery of health care services, such as education of health care professionals, attempts to control administrative costs, and proliferation of high-cost equipment and facilities.

Health insurance purchasing cooperative (HIPC) or health plan purchasing cooperative (HPPC): An organization (typically a nonprofit) that pools individuals or employees to bargain for and purchase coverage from health insurance plans on behalf of individuals and small employers in an attempt to give them the same purchasing clout enjoyed by large employers.

Health maintenance organization (HMO): A type of managed care organization, an HMO is a prepaid health plan that typically provides comprehensive benefits through a network of captive or affiliated providers. Generally only services performed by providers inside the network are covered. The providers may in some cases be salaried staff of the HMO, but typically they are independent doctors, groups, or organizations affiliated with the HMO under a contract.

High-risk pools: State-created insurance pools of individuals with extensive current or anticipated health care needs. These pools spread the risk for those individuals among the health insurance companies doing business in that state. These pools have been used by a number of states in an attempt to extend coverage to their medically uninsurable citizens.

Hospice: An organization that provides services to terminally ill patients and their families with a goal of providing death with dignity. Services may be provided on an inpatient or home care basis and include such things as pain relief, support services, and treatment of symptoms associated with the illness.

Hospitalization plan: A type of indemnity insurance that covers the cost of hospitalization and, in most cases, surgical care, usually up to a predetermined limit. Examples of covered costs include the use of the operating room, radiology services, and hospital room and board. It does not cover outpatient services. Typically, hospital bills are handled on a direct payment basis (the carrier pays the hospital directly). Often there is no deductible and no coinsurance.

Indemnity insurance: The traditional form of insurance in which claims are paid by an insurance company to virtually any provider so long as the services rendered are covered under the policy. Usually the patient pays a deductible. There are different types of indemnity insurance, including hospitalization, major-medical, and comprehensive plans.

Independent practice association (IPA): A group, organized to contract with a managed care organization, consisting of individual physicians or those in small group practices that treat patients from the managed care network as well as private patients.

Individual mandate: A provision included in health care reform legislation that requires individuals to secure and pay for their own health benefits if they are not covered by their employer or eligible for one of the government programs.

Insurance reform: A package of legislative provisions that regulate the marketing practices of health insurance companies. Although various insurance reforms have been considered by Congress, as of this writing none have been enacted. On the other hand, many states have enacted insurance reform legislation. Typically, insurance reforms attempt to address either access to coverage and/or affordability of coverage for the small-group market. (*Compare to* Health care reform.)

Insurance reforms that affect affordability may limit annual premium increases or proscribe that prices fall within certain ranges.

The most notable of the access reforms enacted by the states are the following:

Continuity of coverage: Refers to one or more of the following regulatory provisions: (1) regulations guaranteeing that employers will be able to obtain coverage when they change insurance companies or if their insurer ceases doing business in that market, and/or (2) regulations guaranteeing that employees will be able to obtain new coverage if they change jobs.

Guaranteed issue: A requirement that insurance companies provide coverage to all eligible parties without requiring proof of their insurability.

Guaranteed renewal: A prohibition against canceling insurance policies because of medical histories or including new exclusions at the time of renewal.

Integrated service network (ISN): The state of Minnesota created this type of organization, similar to an HMO but subject to fewer restrictions, to provide the full continuum of health care to specific populations at a predefined cost.

International Classification of Diseases (ICD): A system of classification and diagnoses used to create uniformity in the collection of health information. There have been various versions of ICD, one of which served as the basis for Medicare's diagnosis-related groupings.

Job lock: The phenomenon of people staying in their current jobs because they have an illness or condition (or one of their dependents has an illness or condition) that may make them ineligible for insurance coverage.

Joint Commission on Accreditation of Healthcare Organizations (JCAHO): A body that accredits hospitals and other health care organizations. Some state and federal programs require JCAHO certification as a condition for licensure and participation in government-run health care programs.

Long-term care: Ongoing services, typically associated with care for the elderly, to meet the needs of an individual with a chronic illness or a mental or physical disability. The services may be provided through a home care provider or on an outpatient or inpatient basis, such as through a rehabilitation facility or nursing home.

Major medical insurance: A type of indemnity insurance that provides reimbursement for most medical expenses up to a high maximum benefit and usually subject to coinsurance and deductibles.

Malpractice: Negligent or unprofessional treatment by a service provider that results in injury to the patient.

Managed care: A term that usually is used to describe a type of health care system. In some cases people use the term to also describe the health care management practices employed by managed care organizations or networks.

When describing a system, the term "managed care" refers to a type of health care organization or network, such as a health maintenance organization (HMO), preferred provider organization (PPO), or exclusive provider organization (EPO). As a system, managed care involves a coordinating body (often an insurance company) and a network of providers, such as hospitals, doctors, and other medical personnel.

Managed care may have some health promotion aspects, but at its core it is a health care cost-control mechanism. The most common means employed to control costs are (1) through controlling access, using primary care physicians as gatekeepers to more expensive specialties, and (2) through discounted prices that are prenegotiated between the insurer (coordinating body) and the providers.

Payments to providers may be on a capitated basis, that is, a fixed fee per patient each year regardless of the services that the patient uses.

Managed care organizations or networks are typically organized by insurance companies or provider groups such as hospitals or doctors. In some cases they have been organized by large employers.

Sometimes the term "managed care" will also be used to describe various health care management practices that are typically used by managed care organizations/networks, such as utilization review, case management, or outcome management.

Some managed care networks are "closed panel," which means that participants can only see physicians employed by the plan; "open panel" plans allow participants to see physicians affiliated with the plan as well as those employed by it.

Managed competition: This recently coined term describes a health care system that would bring a different level of competition to the health care market by organizing individuals into purchasing cooperatives and providers into provider networks. Provider networks would then compete for the business of the purchasing cooperatives, with the cooperatives bargaining for the best arrangement for their members.

Mandated benefits: Legislation passed by many states that specifies a minimum set of health benefits that insurance carriers must offer. In a move to make insurance coverage more affordable to small groups, many states have enacted legislation that allows small employers to offer health benefits plans that exclude many of the mandated benefits required in plans offered by larger employers.

Maximum benefit: An absolute limit beyond which an insurer will not pay incurred expenses, even those that were previously eligible to be paid. This limit may apply per case, per year, or for a lifetime.

Medicaid: A government health care program for the poor, with operations and costs shared by the federal and state governments. In 1992 Medicaid covered 31.15 million recipients, with benefit payments totaling $91.48 billion. Medicaid serves less than half of the poverty population (47.2% of the poverty population in 1992). In 1992, some 22.24 million Medicaid recipients were also recipients of Aid to Families with Dependent Children.

Medicaid, along with Medicare, was authorized by federal legislation in 1965 (Public Law 89-97) that took effect in 1966. *See* Health Care Financing Administration (HCFA) which has jurisdiction at the federal level.

Medicaid waiver: Because Medicaid is a costly program for the states and because federal government rules determine eligibility, some states have sought waivers to be able to operate health care programs for the poor under their own rules.

Medical necessity: Health insurance companies often require that hospital stays and other medical treatments be deemed medically necessary before they will agree to cover the costs. Under many plans it is necessary to get advance approval for certain types of care. Deciding that treatment is medically necessary indicates that, without this treatment, the patient's life would be seriously threatened.

Medicare: The federal government health care program for the elderly (those aged 65 and over), financed by payroll taxes, general revenue funds, and some patient premiums. In 1992 Medicare covered 35.58 million recipients, with benefit payments totaling $129.18 billion.

Medicare, along with Medicaid, was authorized by federal legislation in 1965 (Public Law 89-97) that took effect in 1966. *See* Health Care Financing Administration (HCFA), which has jurisdiction at the federal level.

Medicare Part A: The portion of Medicare that is universal, covering hospitalization, home health care, and some skilled nursing facility care.

Medicare Part B: The portion of Medicare that is voluntary, covering outpatient hospital care, partial payment of physician services, and some medical supplies and equipment.

Medigap: Private insurance that supplements Medicare by paying for items not covered by Medicare. Depending on the policy, this may include prescription drugs, deductibles, coinsurance, and other items.

Multiple Employer Welfare Arrangement (MEWA) or Multiple Employer Trust (MET): A legal entity, usually a trust, that results when several unrelated employers combine forces to form a group insurance plan. Some of these plans are self-insured, where the group is responsible for the cost of claims (usually backed up with stop-loss coverage), with administration typically handled by a third-party administrator. Other plans may be fully insured, where the group essentially is a purchasing cooperative that negotiates with an insurance company that is responsible for the cost of the claims and administers the program.

National health care: A health care system that guarantees all citizens a minimum standard of benefits.

Open enrollment: A period of time when individuals can obtain coverage under a group plan without providing proof of their insurability.

Open panel: *See* Managed Care.

Orphan drugs: Refers to drugs covered under the Orphan Drugs Act, a federal law passed in 1983 to encourage development, through tax credits and market rights, of pharmaceuticals for conditions that afflict a limited number of people (under 200,000) and therefore represent a limited and otherwise unprofitable market.

Outcomes management: A patient care system of targeting treatment methods based on the outcome desired, such as discharge within a certain number of days.

Out-of-pocket costs: Expenses that the patient must pay for him/herself, such as the deductible and coinsurance.

Participating physician: A doctor who has agreed to treat the beneficiaries of a particular health insurance plan.

Peer review organization (PRO): Under the Medicare program, an organization that contracts with the HCFA to monitor quality and determine if payments should be made to a provider.

Per diem: A dollar amount set for hospital services (per day) above which the plan will not pay regardless of the cost of those services.

Play-or-pay system: A system of universal coverage where employers are required to assume some responsibility for their employees' health care coverage by doing one of two things: (1) directly providing a plan to employees (play), or (2) paying taxes or payment to a government plan (pay).

Point of service (POS) plan: A health insurance plan that is a hybrid of an indemnity plan and an HMO. A POS varies its share of the payment based on whether the patient uses one of the providers designated by the plan (in which case the plan pays a higher share) or one outside the plan (in which case the plan pays a lower share). The purpose is to give the patient an incentive to use designated providers, which have negotiated with the plan for presumably lower fees than those charged by outside providers.

Portability: The ability of an individual to keep his/her health insurance while he/she is between jobs or moving from one job to another.

Preadmission certification: An evaluation by a health professional, acting on behalf of the insurance carrier, of an attending physician's request to admit a patient to the hospital. The process uses established medical criteria to determine appropriateness and medical necessity of the hospital admission.

Preadmission testing: Many plans require that tests necessary before admission to the hospital be performed on an outpatient basis within a specified number of days before the scheduled admission.

Preexisting condition: A medical condition that an individual has which has been diagnosed prior to obtaining insurance coverage and that the insurer generally takes into account in deciding to provide coverage. Depending on the insurance plan and the type of medical condition, the plan (1) may refuse to cover the individual, (2) may increase its premium, or (3) may refuse to cover the individual for that condition for a certain period of time.

Preferred provider organization (PPO): A health care plan that is similar to an HMO but allows patients to see providers outside of the network, typically with the patient paying a higher share of the cost. PPOs contract with groups of providers who agree to offer the PPO lower fees, typically in exchange for a guaranteed volume of patients and a structure that streamlines the payment process.

Premium: Money paid to an insurance company for coverage.

Premium tax: A tax on the premiums typically collected by a state on premiums paid by policyholders living within its jurisdiction.

Prepaid health plan: A health benefit plan that provides a defined set of health services to an enrolled population for a predetermined premium.

Preventive care: Health care treatments or services designed to keep plan members from becoming sick or to detect the early warning signs of illness. Examples include regular medical, vision, or hearing checkups. Most traditional indemnity plans do not cover these costs, whereas many managed care plans do. Sometimes referred to as *wellness benefits.*

Price controls: A ceiling on prices set by the government, usually though a regulatory agency.

Primary care: General medical care typical of the care provided by routine visits to the doctor.

Prospective payment system: A health care provider payment system associated with Medicare.

Qualified medicare beneficiary: A term associated with Medicare that applies to individuals aged 65 or over with income below the poverty line who are eligible to have the government pay for the costs of Medicare, including Part B premiums, copayments, and deductibles.

Quality assurance: A health care management system that focuses on monitoring patient care and making ongoing improvements to raise the level of quality of care.

Rationing: A method of limiting access to a good or service such as medical care.

Reinsurance: *See* Stop-loss coverage.

Relative value scale (RVS) or resource-based relative value system (RBRVS): The method used by Medicare to reimburse physicians based on the complexity of the treatment or procedure. It was designed to shift care away from high-cost specialists to lower-cost primary physicians.

Risk factors: Conditions that significantly influence one's chances of getting an illness or injury. Common risk factors can include sex, age, race, and family history of health problems. Lifestyle factors, such as smoking, alcohol consumption, or high-fat diet can also be risk factors.

Risk pool: A group of individuals that share common characteristics, such as those that have insurance coverage through the same carrier.

Self-insurance: This term typically refers to an employer's group insurance plan or other type of group plan where the benefits are paid from the resources of the organization rather than by an insurance company. For organized groups, instances of total self-insurance are rare. Typically the group will purchase stop-loss insurance, which provides a ceiling for the costs the group might face, above which the costs are paid by the insurance carrier providing the stop-loss policy.

Self-insurance has become a popular tool with employers to reduce their health benefits costs. Under this arrangement, the employer purchases a group policy with high deductibles and/or high copayments and offers the employee a lower deductible and/or copayment. The employer will self-insure the difference between the high and low deductibles/copayments with the hope that the amount it reimburses to the employees will be lower than the cost associated with buying a higher-cost low-deductible, low-copayment policy.

Single-payer system: A type of health insurance where the government acts as the insurance carrier, collects premium payments, and pays the providers.

Skilled nursing facility: Typically a transition facility for patients between the hospital and home that provides acute care inpatient nursing and rehabilitative services. These services often are covered by Medicare, whereas long-term care is not.

Small-group market: Usually refers to the small-employer market for employee health benefits. Although the term typically refers to employers with fewer than 100 employees, a threshold of 50 employees has been used in some cases.

Stop-loss coverage: Also known as reinsurance, stop-loss coverage is a special type of insurance that self-insuring organizations and health plans purchase as a hedge against unexpected costs.

Typically stop-loss insurance provides a cap on the costs that the plan might incur from any one individual or account. For example, a health plan purchases a stop-loss insurance to cap its cost exposure for any individual at $150,000. If an individual generates more than $150,000 in claims in a year, the stop-loss carrier reimburses the health plan for the amount in excess of $150,000.

Reinsurance, though a specialized type of insurance, is common practice in the insurance industry to minimize risk exposure by spreading the risk across several carriers.

Supplemental insurance: Insurance that provides benefits in addition to a primary insurance policy. For example, retirees may purchase supplemental insurance to help reduce their out-of-pocket expenses for costs not covered by Medicare. To give another example, a family or individual may purchase supplemental insurance to cover services not included in the standard benefits package offered by the employer, such as vision or dental care.

Tax credit: A reduction in amount of taxes owed. A dollar in tax credits yields a dollar in tax savings.

Tax deduction: A reduction in the income that is subject to tax. A dollar of deductions reduces the tax burden by an amount in proportion to the tax rate. For example, a one dollar deduction at a 28% tax rate would yield 28 cents in tax savings.

Tax exclusion: Income that is excluded from taxable compensation. For example, the value of employer-provided health benefits is excluded from the amount of the employee's compensation that is subject to taxes.

Third-party administrator (TPA): A person or organization that handles the administration of a health insurance plan for a group, such as an employer health plan, but does not provide the insurance coverage. TPAs are commonly used by self-insured plans. Since the group is assuming the risk itself rather than involving an insurance company, it needs someone to handle the administrative affairs of the group plan, such as the financial management, payment of claims, etc.

Third-party payer: Health care payments often involve three parties: (1) the patient, (2) the health care provider, and (3) a private insurance company or public insurance program such as Medicare or Medicaid that pays all or part of the bill on behalf of the patient.

Uncompensated care: Health care services provided to a patient that are not paid for, the cost of which is typically spread out over paying patients.

Undercompensated care: Health care services for which the providers are not compensated to a level to meet their cost of providing the care, typically associated with government-run programs. The difference is typically spread out over other patients.

Underinsured: This term refers to people who do not have sufficient insurance coverage to meet their current or anticipated needs. This may include policies that discourage preventive care or those that do not cover needed services.

Underwriting: The process that an insurance company uses to determine the level of risk involved and whether or not to offer to cover that risk, and—if coverage is offered—the premium level that is appropriate to that risk.

Uninsurable risk: A situation where the probability of claims being made or the potential cost of the claim is so great that it does not make business sense for an insurance company to cover that risk.

Uninsured: This term refers to people without health insurance coverage. According to the Census Bureau, in 1992 there were 37.4 million U.S. citizens without health insurance, comprising 14.7% of the population.

Universal coverage: A system of health care that attempts to include all citizens in the country or within a state. Although universal coverage has failed to gain support in Congress, several states have enacted legislation aimed at providing universal coverage to all of their residents.

Usual, customary, and reasonable charges: The cost associated with health care services that is consistent with the going rate for identical or similar services within that geographic area. It is used by insurance carriers to determine the amount to pay health care providers or reimburse policyholders.

Utilization review: A cost- and quality-control process in which health care services provided to the patient are subjected to an independent review. This review may be prospective (prior to the delivery of the services), concurrent, or retrospective (after the services are delivered). The purpose of the review is to determine if services are medically necessary, are delivered in the appropriate setting, and meet predetermined standards of care.

Waiting period: The length of time an employee must wait from his/her date of employment to the date his/her health insurance is effective.

Compiled by Donald Tebbe, January 1995. Some items are reprinted, with permission, from *Glossary of Health Insurance Terms*, published by the Nonprofit Coordinating Committee of New York. Glossary copyright 1995 by the Nonprofit Risk Management Center. Adapted by permission. For more information about the Center's publications and services, visit http://www.nonprofitrisk.org or contact:

Nonprofit Risk Management Center
1001 Connecticut Avenue, NW, Suite 410
Washington, DC 20036
Phone: 202-785-3891
Fax: 202-296-0349

References

Adler, J. (1988). *The client's perception of the working alliance.* Unpublished doctoral dissertation, University of British Columbia, Vancouver, Canada.

Alden, L. E., Wiggins, J. S., & Pincus, A. L. (1990). Construction of circumplex scales for interpersonal problems. *Journal of Personality Assessment, 55,* 521–536.

Bachelor, A. (1991). Comparison and relationship to outcome of diverse dimensions of the helping alliance as seen by client and therapist. *Psychotherapy, 28*(4), 534–549.

Barron, J. W., & Sands, H. (Eds.). (1996). *Impact of managed care on psychodynamic treatment.* Madison, CT: International Universities Press.

Beck, A. T., Epstein, N., Brown, G., & Steer, R. A. (1988). An inventory for measuring clinical anxiety: Psychometric properties. *Journal of Consulting and Clinical Psychology, 56,* 893–897.

Beck, A. T., Steer, R. A., & Brown, R. A. (1996). *Manual for the Beck Depression Inventory–II.* San Antonio, TX: Psychological Corporation.

Beck, A. T., Ward, C. H., Mendelson, M., Mock, J., & Erbaugh, J. (1961). An inventory for measuring depression. *Archives of General Psychiatry, 4,* 561–571.

Bell, M., Billington, R., & Becker, B. (1986). A scale for the assessment of object relations: Reliability, validity, and factorial invariance. *Journal of Clinical Psychology, 42,* 733–741.

Blatt, S. J., D'Afflitti, J. P., & Quinlan, D. M. (1976). Experiences of depression in normal young adults. *Journal of Abnormal Psychology, 85,* 383–389.

Blatt, S. J., D'Afflitti, J. P., & Quinlan, D. M. (1979). *Depressive Experi-*

ences Questionnaire. Unpublished research manual, Yale University, New Haven, CT.

Blatt, S. J., Ford, R. Q., Berman, W., Cook, B., & Meyer, R. (1988). The assessment of change during the intensive treatment of borderline and schizophrenic young adults. *Psychoanalytic Psychology, 5*(2), 127–158.

Blatt, S. J., Quinlan, D. M., Pilkonis, P. A., & Shea, M. T. (1995). Impact of perfectionism and need for approval on the brief treatment of depression: The National Institute of Mental Health treatment of depression collaborative research program revisited. *Journal of Consulting and Clinical Psychology, 63*(1), 125–132.

Blatt, S. J., Wiseman, H., Prince-Gibson, E., & Gatt, C. (1991). Object representations and change in clinical functioning. *Psychotherapy, 28*(2), 273–283.

Blatt, S. J., Zohar, A. H., Quinlan, D. M., Zuroff, D. C., & Mongrain, M. (1995). Subscales within the dependency factor of the Depressive Experience Questionnaire. *Journal of Personality Assessment, 64*(2), 319–339.

Bloom, B. L. (1992). *Planned short-term psychotherapy.* Boston: Allyn & Bacon.

Bollas, C., & Sundelson, D. (1996). *The new informants: The betrayal of confidentiality in psychoanalysis and psychotherapy.* Northvale, NJ: Aronson.

Bongar, B., & Beutler, L. E. (1995). *Comprehensive textbook of psychotherapy: Theory and practice.* New York: Oxford University Press.

Bordin, E. S. (1979). The generalizability of the psychoanalytic concept of the working alliance. *Psychotherapy: Theory, Research and Practice, 16*(3), 252–260.

Butcher, J. N., Dahlstrom, W. G., Graham, J. R., Tellegen, A., & Kaemmer, B. (1989). *Minnesota Multiphasic Personality Inventory (MMPI-II). Manual for administration and scoring.* Minneapolis: University of Minnesota Press.

Cattell, R. B. (1966). Patterns of change: Measurement in relation to state-dimension, trait change, lability, and process concepts. *Handbook of multivariate experimental psychology.* Chicago: Rand McNally.

Craig, R. J. (1993). *Psychological assessment with the Millon Clinical Multiaxial Inventory: An interpretive guide.* Odessa, FL: Psychological Assessment Resources.

Craighead, L. W., Craighead, W. E., Kazdin, L., & Mahoney, M. J. (1994). *Cognitive and behavioral interventions: An empirical approach to mental health problems.* Boston: Allyn & Bacon.

Dana, R. H., Conner, M. G., & Allen, J. (1996). Quality of care and cost-containment in managed mental health: Policy, education, research, advocacy. *Psychological Reports, 79,* 1395–1422.

Derogatis, L. R. (1975). *SCL-90-R: Administration, scoring, and procedural manual.* Baltimore: Clinical Psychometric Research.

Derogatis, L. R. (1993). *Brief Symptom Inventory.* Minneapolis, MN: National Computer Systems.

Derogatis, L. R., & Melisaratos, N. (1983). The Brief Symptom Inventory: An introductory report. *Psychological Medicine, 13,* 595–605.

DeRubeis, R. J., & Feeley, M. (1990). Determinants of change in cognitive therapy for depression. *Cognitive Therapy and Research, 14*(5), 469–482.

Drummond, H. E., Ghosh, S., Ferguson, A., Brackenridge, D., & Tiplady, B. (1995). Electronic quality of life questionnaires: A comparison of pen-based electronic questionnaires with conventional paper in a gastrointestinal study. *Quality of Life Research, 4*(1), 21–26.

Endicott, J., Spitzer, R., Fleiss, J. L., & Cohen, J. (1976). The Global Assessment Scale: A procedure for measuring the overall severity of psychiatric disturbance. *Archives of General Psychiatry, 33,* 766–771.

Feldman, L. A. (1993). Distinguishing depression and anxiety in self-report: Evidence from confirmatory factor analysis on nonclinical and clinical samples. *Journal of Consulting and Clinical Psychology, 61*(4), 631–638.

Fishler, P., Sperling, M. B., & Carr, A. (1990). Assessment of adult relatedness: A review of empirical findings from object relations and attachment theory. *Journal of Personality Assessment, 55*(3&4), 499–520.

Franche, R. L., & Dobson, K. S. (1992). Self-criticism and interpersonal dependency as vulnerability factors to depression. *Cognitive Therapy and Research, 16*(4), 419–435.

Frank, A. F., & Gunderson, J. G. (1990). The role of the therapeutic alliance in the treatment of schizophrenia. *Archives of General Psychiatry, 47,* 228–236.

Frieswyk, S. H., Allen, J. G., Colson, D. B., Coyne, L., Gabbard, G. O., Horwitz, L., & Newsom, G. (1986). Therapeutic alliance: Its place as an outcome variable in dynamic psychotherapy research. *Journal of Consulting and Clinical Psychology, 1,* 32–39.

Frisch, M. (1994). *Quality of Life Inventory.* Minneapolis, MN: National Computer Systems.

Gaston, L., Marmar, C. R., Thompson, L. W., & Gallagher, D. (1988). Relation of patient pretreatment characteristics to the therapeutic alliance in diverse psychotherapies. *Journal of Consulting and Clinical Psychology, 56,* 483–489.

Gaudry, E., Spielberger, C. D., & Vagg, P. R. (1975). Validation of the state–trait distinction in anxiety research. *Multivariate Behavior Research, 10*, 331–341.

Grundy, C. T., Lunnen, K. M., Lambert, M. J., Ashton, J. E., & Tovey, D. R. (1994). The Hamilton Rating Scale for Depression: One scale or many? *Clinical Psychology: Science and Practice, 1*(2), 197–205.

Hamilton, M. (1960). A rating scale for depression. *Journal of Neurology, Neurosurgery, and Psychiatry, 23*, 56–61.

Hartley, D. (1985). Research on the therapeutic alliance in psychotherapy. In R. Hales & A. Frances (Eds.), *Psychiatry update annual review* (pp. 532–549). Washington, DC: American Psychiatric Press.

Hazan, C., & Shaver, P. (1987). Romantic love conceptualized as an attachment process. *Journal of Personality and Social Psychology, 52*(3), 511–524.

Horowitz, L. M., Rosenberg, S. E., Bauer, B. A., Ureno, G., & Villasenor, V. S. (1988). Inventory of Interpersonal Problems: Psychometric properties and clinical applications. *Journal of Consulting and Clinical Psychology, 56*, 885–892.

Horvath, A. O., & Luborsky, L. (1993). The role of therapeutic alliance in psychotherapy. *Journal of Consulting and Clinical Psychology, 61*, 561–573.

Horvath, A. O., & Symonds, D. B. (1991). Relation between working alliance and outcome in psychotherapy: A meta-analysis. *Journal of Counseling Psychology, 38*, 139–149.

Ihilevich, D., & Gleser, G. C. (1986). *Defense mechanisms. Their classification, correlates, and measurement with the Defense Mechanism Inventory.* Owosso, MI: DMI Associates.

Kazdin, A. E. (1994). Methodology, design, and evaluation in psychotherapy research. In A. E. Bergin & S. L. Garfield (Eds.), *Handbook of psychotherapy and behavior change* (4th ed., pp. 19–71). New York: Wiley.

Koss, M. P., & Shiang, J. (1994). Research on brief psychotherapy. In A. E. Bergin & S. L. Garfield (Eds.), *Handbook of psychotherapy and behavior change* (pp. 664–700). New York: Wiley.

Lambert, M. J., Hatch, D. R., Kingston, M. D., & Edwards, B. C. (1986). Zung, Beck, and Hamilton rating scales as measures of treatment outcome: A meta-analytic comparison. *Journal of Consulting and Clinical Psychology, 54*, 54–59.

Lazar, S. G. (Ed.). (1997). *Extended dynamic psychotherapy: Making the case in an era of managed care.* (Supplement to *Psychoanalytic Inquiry.*) Hillsdale, NJ: Analytic Press.

Luborsky, L. (1962). Clinician's judgment of mental health: A proposed scale. *Archives of General Psychiatry, 7*, 407–417.

Luborsky, L., & Auerbach, A. (1985). The therapeutic relationship in psychodynamic psychotherapy: The research evidence and its meaning for practice. In R. Hales & A. Frances (Eds.), *Psychiatry update annual review* (pp. 550–561). Washington, DC: American Psychiatric Press.

Luborsky, L., McLellan, A. T., Woody, G. E., O'Brien, C. P., & Auerbach, A. (1985). Therapist success and its determinants. *Archives of General Psychiatry, 42,* 602–611.

Malan, D. H. (1976). *The frontier of brief psychotherapy.* New York: Plenum.

Marmar, C. R., Weiss, D. S., & Gaston, L. (1989). Toward the validation of the California therapeutic alliance rating system. *Psychological Assessment, 1*(1), 46–52.

McHorney, C. A., Ware, J. E., & Raczek, A. E. (1993). The MOS 36-Item Short Form Health Survey (SF-36): II. Psychometric and clinical tests of validity in measuring physical and mental health constructs. *Medical Care, 31*(3), 247–263.

Miller, I. J. (1996). Managed care is harmful to outpatient mental health services: A call for accountability. *Professional Psychology: Research and Practice, 27*(4), 349–363.

Millon, T. (1989). *Manual for the MCMI-II* (2nd ed.). Minneapolis, MN: National Computer Systems.

Moore, B. E., & Fine, B. D. (1990). *Psychoanalytic terms and concepts.* New Haven, CT: Yale University Press.

Moras, K., & Strupp, H. H. (1982). Pretherapy interpersonal relations, patients' alliance and the outcome in brief therapy. *Archives of General Psychiatry, 39,* 405–409.

Morey, L. C. (1991). *Personality Assessment Inventory.* Odessa, FL: Psychological Assessment Resources.

Morin, C. M., & Colecchi, C. A. (1995). Psychological assessment of older adults. In J. N. Butcher (Ed.), *Clinical personality assessment: Practical approaches* (pp. 172–191). New York: Oxford University Press.

Noble, H. (1995, July 3). Quality is focus for health plans. *New York Times,* 1.

Overholser, J. C., & Freiheit, S. R. (1994). Assessment of interpersonal dependency using the Millon Clinical Multiaxial Inventory–II (MCMI-II) and the Depressive Experience Questionnaire. *Personality and Individual Differences, 17*(1), 71–78.

Perry, J. C. (1993). Defenses and their effects. In N. E. Miller, L. Luborsky, J. P. Barber, & J. P. Docherty (Eds.), *Psychodynamic treatment research: A handbook for clinical practice* (pp. 274–306). New York: Basic Books.

Perry, J. C., & Cooper, S. H. (1989). An empirical study of defense mechanisms: I. Clinical interview and life vignette ratings. *Archives of General Psychiatry, 46,* 444–452.

Piper, W. E., Azim, H. F. A., Joyce, A. S., McCallum, M., Nixon, G. W. H., & Segal, P. S. (1991). Quality of object relations vs. interpersonal functioning as predictor of therapeutic alliance and psychotherapy outcome. *Journal of Nervous and Mental Disease, 179,* 432–438.

Pollack, W. S. (1996). The survival of psychoanalytic psychotherapy in managed care: "Reports of my death are greatly exaggerated." In J. W. Barron & H. Sands (Eds.), *Impact of managed care on psychodynamic treatment* (pp. 107–129). Madison, CT: International Universities Press.

Raue, P. J., Castunguay, L. G., & Goldfried, M. R. (1991). *The working alliance: A comparison of two therapies.* Paper presented at the annual meeting of the Society of Psychotherapy Integration, London.

Rounsaville, B. J., Chevron, E. S., Prusoff, B. A., Elkin, I., Imber, S., Sotsky, S., & Watkins, J. (1987). The relation between specific and general dimensions of the psychotherapy process in interpersonal psychotherapy of depression. *Journal of Consulting and Clinical Psychology, 55,* 379–384.

Sack, A., Sperling, M. B., Fagen, G., & Foelsch, P. (1996). Attachment style, history, and behavioral contrasts for a borderline and normal sample. *Journal of Personality Disorders, 10*(1), 88–102.

Safran, J. D., & Wallner, L. K. (1991). The relative predictive validity of two therapeutic measures in cognitive therapy. *Psychological Assessment, 3*(2), 188–195.

Seligman, M. E. P., & Levant, R. F. (1998). Managed care policies rely on inadequate science. *Professional Psychology, 29*(3), 211–212.

Small, R. F., & Barnhill, L. R. (Eds.). (1998). *Practicing in the new mental health marketplace: Ethical, legal, and moral issues.* Washington, DC: American Psychological Association.

Sperling, M. B., & Berman, W. H. (1991). An attachment classification of desperate love. *Journal of Personality Assessment, 56,* 45–55.

Sperling, M. B., Foelsch, P., & Grace, C. (1996). Measuring adult attachment: Are self-report instruments congruent? *Journal of Personality Assessment, 67*(1), 37–51.

Sperling, M. B., & Lyons, L. (1994). Representations of attachment and psychotherapeutic change. In M. B. Sperling & W. H. Berman, *Attachment in adults: Clinical and developmental perspectives* (pp. 331–347). New York: Guilford Press.

Spielberger, C. D. (1983). *Manual for the State–Trait Anxiety Inventory (Form Y)*. Palo Alto, CA: Consulting Psychologists Press.

Spielberger, C. D. (1989). *State–Trait Anxiety Inventory: A comprehensive bibliography* (2nd ed.). Palo Alto, CA: Consulting Psychologists Press.

Spielberger, C. D., Gorsuch, R. L., & Lushene, R. D. (1970). *STAI: Manual for the State–Trait Anxiety Inventory*. Palo Alto, CA: Consulting Psychologists Press.

Spielberger, C. D., Ritterband, L. M., Sydeman, S. J., Reheiser, E. C., & Unger, K. K. (1995). Assessment of emotional states and personality traits: Measuring psychological vital signs. In J. N. Butcher (Ed.), *Clinical personality assessment: Practical approaches* (pp. 42–58). New York: Oxford University Press.

Terranova, R., McGrath, R. E., & Pogge, D. (1999, March). Another look at short forms: High-point code convergence for the MMPI-2. Presented at the midwinter meeting of the Society for Personality Assessment, New Orleans, LA.

Walrond-Skinner, S. (1986). *Dictionary of psychotherapy*. London: Routledge & Kegan Paul.

Ware, J. E., & Sherbourne, C. D. (1992). The MOS 36-Item Short-Form Health Survey (SF-36). *Medical Care, 30*(6), 473–483.

Weissman, M. M., & Bothwell, S. (1976). Assessment of social adjustment by patient self-report. *Archives of General Psychiatry, 33,* 1111–1115.

Williams, J. B. (1988). Structured interview guides for the Hamilton Rating Scales. *Archives of General Psychiatry, 45,* 742–747.

Index

160